Contents

About the author

Fiona Marshall has written widely on health and psychology. She is the author of ten books, seven of them for Sheldon Press, and also a novel.

Author's note to the reader

This is not a medical book and is not intended to replace advice from your doctor. Consult your pharmacist or doctor if you believe you have any of the symptoms described, and if you think you might need medical help.

Introduction: the message of tiredness

For three years I commuted into London on the 6.37a.m. Every morning, you could look down the length of the train and see that every single seat on those 12 carriages was taken, and that most of the travellers were asleep. They were quite uninhibited sleepers. Mouths open and heads dropped back, they snored openly; their heads nodded downward and sideways; occasionally someone would demonstrate the soundness of this sleep by tumbling right off the seat into the aisle. Once, I even saw a couple of labourers, unable to get a seat, lying full length by the doors in their boots. The train had become a moving bed. These commuters weren't just indulging in a little nap. This was serious sleep, of the depth and freedom you usually associate with your own bed. On winter mornings, with the train rushing through the dark countryside, one had the impression that the driver was the only person awake on the entire train.

Tiredness is the epidemic of today. We're all exhausted – not just shift workers, politicians and young mothers, but everyone. Too tired to socialize, too tired to talk on the phone, too tired to make love, too tired to cook. At any given time, one in four people feels unusually tired, and one in 10 have prolonged fatigue. It's likely that many more people just put up with it and don't seek help. Women are more likely to be affected than men, although I must say I have rarely seen so many men sleeping so deeply as I did on that early-morning train.

So why is 'feeling tired' one of the most common reasons for consulting the doctor? Is tiredness the inevitable result of today's lifestyle, in which the immune system takes a battering from the deadly quartet of constant stress, long work hours, poor diet and lack of exercise? Has our consumer society merely dispensed with down-time as unproductive? This certainly isn't how nature works. Look around and you will see that dormancy is a vital part of the natural ebb and flow of nature. Think of the Latin word *dormire*, 'to sleep'. Dormancy allows the natural world to rest and regroup. Temperate climate plants need dormancy – experiments have shown that an eternal summer is usually fatal to deciduous plants, and some seeds need to pass through a phase of intense cold in order to flourish. Freezing cold also kills disease-causing micro-organisms and weaker plant specimens, assuring the survival of the stronger and continuation of the species. Freezing also cracks the top layers of earth, breaking the soil up and so opening the way for new, different plants to grow in the coming year. There is no spring without winter. Equally, humans need balance. A time to rest, a time in which to do nothing.

In today's busy society, we often ignore this need for deep, natural – and apparently useless – rest. We see the results in the doctor's surgery: shattered people hoping for a magic medical pick-me-up. Often, though, doctors can find no physical cause, and so no cure for tiredness. Sleep deprivation and overwork are two main reasons held by the conventional medical view to be responsible for tiredness, in the absence of a physical cause such as anaemia, thyroid problems or heart disease. Other conditions linked with tiredness are slowly making their way into the medical canon, including chronic fatigue syndrome, fibromyalgia and, perhaps less reliably, candidiasis. These relatively new conditions – chronic fatigue syndrome, for example, was first defined by a panel of international experts in 1994 – still meet with plenty of misunderstanding, not to say opposition, from the medical profession and general public alike, some of whom persist in viewing them as dubious refuges for malingerers and the mentally ill. This view is, however, gradually dispersing under increasing emphasis on the physical aspects of these conditions.

While this book gives some basic information about chronic fatigue syndrome, it is not specifically about this, although I hope it may prove useful to anyone who has that condition or a similar one. (For an approach aimed at managing the symptoms of chronic fatigue syndrome, read *Coping with Chronic Fatigue* by Trudie Chalder, Sheldon Press, 2002.) This book's main emphasis is on the walking weary, those who are healthy and getting on with their lives but are inexplicably tired – the many who, after much thought, troop to the doctor in a last-ditch attempt to help them with their fatigue, only to come home without a diagnosis, and with an apparently clean bill of health. It is also for those who don't bother going to their GP, because they feel it's nobler to struggle on alone, or perhaps because they feel they're not going to get the help they need there. In other words, this book is for the person who feels 'tired all the time' without a defined medical condition, using 'tiredness' and 'fatigue' interchangeably as general words.

Tiredness is a message that should never be ignored. It is not acceptable or natural to feel tired all the time if you are healthy and have had enough water, food and sleep. Neither is persistent tiredness an inevitable consequence of growing older or modern life. Tiredness should never be accepted as 'one of those things' or viewed as something you have to learn to live with. Whether it's down to insomnia, trying to be in three places at once, diabetes or sheer boredom, tiredness is the body's way of signalling that it has had enough, and that something needs to change. Persistent tiredness should always be taken seriously.

It is hoped that this book will help you with the process of tackling your tiredness, although you should see your doctor first to check for any physical causes for it. Once you have the all-clear in terms of health, other main areas to consider are lifestyle and sleep, which are covered in Chapters 5 and 8, respectively. The role of stress, and in particular the stress hormones, is a vital one in fatigue – some think it is at the heart of chronic fatigue syndrome itself – and is discussed in Chapter 6, followed by the female hormones in Chapter 7.

Chapter 9 considers the central role of nutrition, and Chapter 10 the importance of activity and exercise.

As you can see, no one approach is suggested as a miracle cure for tiredness; just as there tends to be no single cause, so there is no single treatment – if there were, we'd all know about it and it would be the subject of this book! Many people do become frustrated with their tiredness when it fails to yield to single-strategy treatments, such as a change of diet, and so it's worth bearing in mind that tiredness may well yield to a range of approaches.

Finally, contradictory though it may seem, it isn't perhaps always appreciated that there may be a price to pay for giving up tiredness. It may mean giving up other things – status, money, activities, stimulation, habit. The habit of eating the same foods, doing the same amount of exercise, even the habit of rushing into work, and back, at the same time every day. Tiredness can also sometimes mask other problems we may not want to face, such as dissatisfaction with job or living arrangements. Cure the tiredness, and we may have to make the effort of changing situations that, at the moment, we just don't have the energy to deal with.

Tiredness challenges us to break those habits, to come out of the comfort zone. And it's wise to try, because tiredness is cumulative. Left to run on unchecked, it threatens quality of life, safety and health itself. It can move from gentle hints to sledgehammer techniques, as the survivor of any fatigue-related accident can tell you.

As well as being a factor in 20–30 per cent of road traffic accidents, long-term tiredness may affect your immune system and make you prone to illnesses such as heart disease, digestive disorders, abdominal pains and hormonal imbalances. Research has also suggested that sleep loss may increase the risk of obesity because chemicals and hormones that play a key role in controlling appetite are released during sleep.

Less dramatically, perhaps one of the real dangers of tiredness is that we become acclimatized to it; we gradually accept the more limited perspective it imposes, and even begin to forget what life was like in the energy-filled days. Indeed, the tiredness itself stops us protesting too much at the diminution in our quality of life; we soldier on. Until, that is, we become ill, or just too tired to continue with plans and projects we really do care about.

The good news is that it is possible to get that precious energy back – although perhaps not as much as you'd like. This book is also about being realistic and realizing that energy can't always be manufactured to keep up with the demands of your average superwoman or superman. It is, however, possible to restore enough energy for an averagely busy life – and a little more. It is possible to build energy so that you have some in reserve.

Adequate energy doesn't mean putting off shopping or putting off meeting a friend because you're 'too tired'; nor does it mean being overwhelmed by the morning tasks of breakfast and dressing, which can reduce a really tired person to tears; it doesn't mean dragging through life, or just surviving. Adequate energy means getting into work with reasonable ease, enjoying the day rather than not, and having a little energy to spare at the end of it. It means having the ability to sort stresses out in a considered way, rather than reacting to every buffet that comes along. It means having the energy to go swimming or walking with your family when you want to, instead of being the one left at home while your partner takes the children out again. It means making time and energy for what *you* want to do in life, with a deep sense of wellbeing. It is hoped that this book will help you towards this desirable state.

How to use this book and beat fatigue

1 Eliminate easily detectable physical problems – *see your doctor.*
   Among the most common causes of fatigue are anaemia; thyroid
   problems; any chronic disease affecting the heart, kidneys, gut
   and other organs; and depression (see Chapters 2–4).
2 Tackle any sleep problems (see Chapter 8).
3 Look at your lifestyle, level of activity and stress – overwork and
   doing too much are other common, often denied main causes of
   tiredness (see Chapters 5 and 6).
4 Examine your diet. You will probably benefit from eliminating
   sugar, alcohol and white flour, and from consuming more fresh
   fruit and vegetables and more foods that are rich in vitamin C, the
   B vitamins, essential fatty acid and magnesium (see Chapter 9).
5 Gradually build more activity and exercise into your life (see
   Chapter 10) and see whether any complementary remedies might
   help (see Chapter 11).
6 Some people may need to consider whether they have chronic
   fatigue syndrome or other fatigue-related conditions (see
   Chapter 12).
7 Take it step by step, and give it time. Tiredness is cumulative. Bear
   in mind that it has probably taken you years to become so tired,
   and so it may take a while to feel better.
8 If you don't experience improvement after three months, visit
   your doctor again and perhaps get a second opinion.

1

How tired are you?

What is tiredness trying to tell you? Persistent mild fatigue is usually considered a reaction to lack of sleep or to working too hard and too long, and it's true that these are two major causes of fatigue. But tiredness can also be shouting loud and clear about your health, your boredom levels and your stress load.

The context of tiredness certainly bears examining, and part of today's widespread tiredness is thought to be due to our heavy work culture. Despite the introduction of the European Working Time Directive, which attempts to limit the working week to a maximum of 48 hours, working hours are in practice longer. A study conducted by the Trades Union Congress (TUC) showed that that more than four million of us regularly spend more time than that at the workplace. The rest of us are working an average of 43.6 hours at work each week – equivalent to an extra three whole days every month. As a nation we are now spending more time at work than anyone else in Europe.

It is even possible to die of overwork, at least in Japan, where *karoshi* ('death from overwork', also known as 'salary sudden death syndrome') has been causing concern since the 1970s following a surge in sudden deaths of several high-ranking executives (usually from heart attack or stroke precipitated by stress.)

Further studies confirm how exhausted we are. A survey of 5,000 people by Legal and General found that lack of sleep was the biggest health concern for 42 per cent of those questioned, followed by fatigue for 34 per cent. Stress and depression were other concerns. It was concluded that working long hours combined with not seeing enough of friends and family is a threat to our health.

The Chartered Management Institute report *Quality of Working Life* showed that more than half of us experience feelings of constant tiredness at work, and even more of us suffer from insomnia. Research from the Chartered Institute of Personnel and Development also revealed that people married to their job find that, while 'workaholism' or intense work commitment puts a strain on relationships, partners tend to tolerate the situation, possibly because of what survey author Melissa Compton-Edwards calls the 'Faustian pact' of long working hours in return for a decent standard of living.

Globalization and technology also conspire to blur the separation between private and public life in our corporate-technological civilization. Online access, email and mobile phones ensure we can work not just in the office but also at home or on the road (if not asleep); even when such technology concerns only our leisure, it can still be very disruptive – as in, 'I'll just send an email.'

The media megaphone, never switched off, also ensures that we are fed a constant undercurrent of anxieties that keep us engaged, at least superficially, with events we can do nothing about, contributing to a low-level, free-ranging anxiety. Sleep problems have spiralled. It seems as though we never really allow ourselves to switch off completely – there is always something else to be done looming on the horizon, whether you're a mother at home, a worker with a part-time job or a full-powered career person. To relax – really relax – becomes a numinous event.

The problem is that energy is not infinite but has a natural ebb and flow, which technology and work hours often over-ride. This isn't to demand a return to days when we all chopped our own wood and dug our own wells, although this does suit some people. But it is to say that energy and health are not resources by right; indeed, there are times when they seem like privileges that must be earned by attentive care. Tiredness presents one of these times.

Women are particularly vulnerable to tiredness. A typically tired person is a woman with two or more children, who has regular periods and so is at risk of anaemia, who's also working and maybe has the care of elderly parents to think about as well. She may not have time to shop and cook proper meals, and will almost certainly skimp on sleep and rest. Women may be quite adept at ignoring tiredness while they continue multi-tasking – for a while. However, over a period of time fatigue builds up until it can no longer be disregarded. Often, by the time women get round to acknowledging their tiredness, it has built up to proportions that can no longer be disregarded; they do something about it because they have to.

For example, Lucy was a busy mother of two who worked as a part-time librarian. She could just about manage until her elderly mother came to live with them. Always noted for her speed and efficiency, Lucy now found she was 'slowing down' drastically. Tasks that had previously been routine, like washing up in the mornings, now became a huge chore. Lucy couldn't work out why she had become so slow, so incompetent, so – well, so tired.

There may be other signs and symptoms such as weight gain, depression or acute pre-menstrual syndrome (see below).

Of course, men tire too, and may equally be poor at admitting fatigue. It's just not done for men to be tired in today's society; although mores dictate that they may be able to get away with it more in a domestic situation. At home, men may be better at getting the extra rest they need in their leisure time – often, they're the ones with their feet up in front of the TV while the woman is catching up on the housework or shopping at week-ends. Not always, though.

For example, Paul was an environmental biologist who worked from home, and cared for his three young children, taking them to and from school and nursery, making tea, organizing sports and other activities for them, and generally leading a life of non-stop activity. His wife had a high-powered job in the city. Friends noted that, while Paul adored his kids and loved his chosen life-style, he had aged visibly under this gruelling routine and had put on quite a bit of weight. His woes culminated in an attack of acute appendicitis with complications, and he was told by his doctors to take it easy for quite a long time.

Anyone can be vulnerable to this kind of engrained tired-ness – not the natural kind that vanishes after a good night's sleep, but an insidious, cumulative condition that may first destroy quality of life, and then health itself.

Symptoms

If you feel tired, surely you feel, well, tired? In fact, tiredness can manifest as a range of symptoms. In the early stages of tiredness these may come and go, but unless action is taken, tiredness tends to persist, and symptoms may last for longer and longer.

They include:

- feeling utterly exhausted, so that you have to go and put your feet up;
- feeling mentally exhausted, 'blah' or used up – you just want to withdraw from everyone and hide away in a space of your own;
- being tired in the morning, even after a full night's sleep;
- feeling you've lost the ability to bounce back from stress, and taking setbacks too seriously;
- being rundown or going down with minor illnesses more often;
- headaches;
- 'achiness' or joint pain, feeling unwell, feeling 'fluey';
- poor short-term memory and concentration, confusion, irritability;

- food cravings, especially for sweets, carbohydrates and, some-times, salty snacks;
- a reliance on caffeine to get you through the day;
- a reliance on alcohol for a 'lift' in the evening;
- loss of motivation;
- difficulty in making decisions;
- slowness at routine tasks – they used to take much less time;
- feelings of depression and sadness – crying ('I'm just so tired I can't cope').

Some of these symptoms may be relevant to other conditions, such as fibromyalgia ('achiness') or depression (lack of motiva-tion). The tired person may not have all of these symptoms, but the list does show that tiredness can sometimes masquerade as other complaints (such as headaches.)

So how do you begin to help yourself? The first step is working out how tired you are. This may seem a bit quixotic to some – surely if you're tired, you're tired! However, there's no doubt that it's easier to tackle mild fatigue than severe fatigue, and it can be useful to be able to define your tiredness if you do want to explain your condition to your doctor. It may also help you to be more aware of unusual fatigue (over and above the normal, run-of-the-mill, get-through-the-day tiredness), which may signal a health disorder.

Categories of tiredness

As tiredness can mean different things to different people, it may help you to know that doctors tend to group fatigue into three broad groups, to help them to understand what someone means when they say they are 'tired':

- lack of energy (the main type);
- lack of drive;
- lack of wakefulness.

Lack of energy

The majority of people who say that they are persistently fatigued mean that they don't have enough energy to get through some, many or all of the tasks of daily living. This can mean anything from being exhausted by the end of a busy day to being worn out by brushing their teeth, or anywhere in between. This sort of tiredness feels as if your batteries have run down, and it is what the bulk of this book is about.

Tiredness of this type can come from a very wide range of potential causes. Anaemia (lack of blood), diabetes, abnormal activity of the thyroid gland, kidney failure and some types of infection are just a few of the 'physical' causes that a doctor may spot fairly easily from clinical examination and preliminary blood tests. Feeling tired must be distinguished from feeling breathless, although the two may coexist, because breathlessness raises a whole extra series of possibilities to do mainly with the condition of the heart and lungs.

Lack of drive

Lack of drive, lack of motivation or lack interest in life are among the main symptoms of depression. Additional symptoms apart from low mood include feelings of guilt, feelings of hopelessness, poor sleep, changes in appetite, lack of interest in sex, lack of confidence and self-esteem, lack of tolerance and thoughts of suicide. Tiredness is something that is often complained about by someone who is depressed. Depression can take all sorts of less obvious forms. It might be, for example, the real reason why someone has been losing weight, or has intractable back pain. Feelings of anxiety commonly coexist with depression, often have the same underlying causes and may respond to the same sorts of treatment (see Chapter 4).

A lack of drive can also frequently come from trying to cope with the many stresses and strains of daily life (see Chapter 5).

Lack of wakefulness

A tendency to fall asleep too easily, in inappropriate circumstances, is the underlying cause of fatigue in a minority of people, although the numbers affected are on the increase. A wide range of causes can be behind this, including excessive sedation from drugs (prescribed or otherwise), excess alcohol intake or a condition called sleep apnoea (see Chapter 11).

Bear in mind that these categories are useful in guiding you to an awareness of the nature of your tiredness, but they are also limited, so don't be too rigid about any definitions. They may also overlap – for example, there is no reason why someone with fatigue may not also be depressed, or become so after a period of time feeling ill.

Tiredness test

The test below gives another way to assess how tired you are and how tiredness may be affecting your life.

A: How often do you wake up feeling tired?
1: Less than once a week
2: Up to three times a week
3: Most days
4: I never feel rested after sleeping

B: How much of an effort can it be to get out of bed?
1: It's not a problem
2: Some days it can be difficult to get going
3: It usually takes a big effort
4: Without help I would have to stay in bed

C: How often do you need to rest?
1: Hardly ever
2: Only after brisk exercise
3: Regularly, even without doing much
4: It seems as if I'm always having to rest

D: Has tiredness made it hard for you to be sociable?
1: Not significantly
2: Now and again I've had to bow out of engagements
3: A lot of the time I haven't got the energy to keep up with family or friends
4: It's a very long time since I was last able to go out or do what I liked

E: Has being tired had any impact on personal relationships?
1: I don't have any significant problems in that area
2: Being tired can cause difficulties occasionally but we cope
3: My lack of energy is causing friction with my partner, family or friends

F: Has tiredness had any impact on your employability?
1: No
2: I've had to make some adjustments but have been able to keep working
3: I've had to take a lot of sick leave, and this is causing increasing difficulty
4: I've lost my job or could not get a job in my present state

G: What is your present view of how tiredness affects your life?
1: It's not really bothering me that much
2: It if gets no worse than this I can find ways to cope
3: I'm struggling with it
4: Tiredness is the number one problem in my life

Your results

There were seven questions. Take the number of each response and add the numbers up. Any score over 7 indicates that fatigue has at least some degree of importance to your life.

5–7: You experience a normal degree of tiredness when appropriate but fatigue isn't a problem.
8–10: You seem to be not too badly affected and are generally coping with the problems that fatigue causes.
11–14: Fatigue has quite a big impact on you, and although there are lots of bad days, they are about balanced by the good ones.
15–21: Fatigue is a major issue for you and is having a significant impact on how you interact with other people and the world around you.
22–28: You are severely affected by fatigue. Hopefully, the advice in this book will help to reduce the difficulties you are experiencing.

2

Am I ill?

This is often the secret – or not so secret – worry that underlies persistent tiredness. What does it mean when I am too tired to go out as planned, when I get through a day at work punch-drunk, when I come home from the shops exhausted? Well, first and foremost, it means you're tired, and often justly so.

The right to be tired is often overlooked in our society. Indeed, there are times when people *should* be tired. Fighting your way round a packed supermarket is exhausting, doing a day's work may use up all your energy, the commute home on an over-crowded tube is draining, and it's natural to feel too tired to go out at the end of a really busy day. Tiredness is the body's way of crying out for rest. It is possible, then, to be unduly alarmed at what is after all natural tiredness, or to over-diagnose tiredness. Some tiredness is inevitable in every life.

Many people, however, worry that some kind of illness underlies their inability to muster enough energy to meet life's demands. The good news is that if you have been to your doctor and been thoroughly checked out – which may take time and require return visits – you are unlikely to be suffering from a missed diagnosis of a very rare disease. Only a minority of people are found to have a physical or organic cause for their fatigue – some 10 per cent. However, many people feel that an organic cause ought to be discovered for their tiredness.

This is where we may run into trouble with the doctor.

Classical medical training is disease-biased: tiredness is a symptom, not a disease

Part of the patient–doctor tussle over persistent fatigue is the search for an identifiable physical cause for tiredness, which is all too often elusive. Traditionally, doctors do take a more objective, reductive approach to tiredness because they have to – tiredness alone isn't usually enough for a diagnosis – while patients think more in terms of the quality and experience of their own tiredness, with the context and nature of tiredness being different for different people. We know, however, that the classic dualistic mind–body split is, for most tired people, a waste of time, because it doesn't result in help – and help is usually what tired people need. For practical, recovery purposes, it appears that management is more important than the cause, especially if, as seems likely, persistent fatigue is caused by a combination of factors and chronic fatigue represents the extreme end of natural, everyday tiredness.

One reason why conventional medicine may be of limited help with tiredness is because of the split in standard medical thinking between 'illnesses of the mind' and 'illnesses of the body' – a split that is almost useless in many cases of tiredness.

Doctors tend first to look for a physical – organic – cause for tiredness. Go to your doctor with tiredness, and you are likely to be – indeed you should be – tested for underlying conditions such as anaemia, thyroid problems and diabetes. Tiredness itself is a symptom, not a disease. A doctor's job is to diagnose disease, and to identify the pathology or disease mechanism that causes it.

While blood and other tests will sometimes highlight a real physical problem that can be treated, more often the tests come back normal, and people leave the surgery feeling they are back to square one.

As tiredness is not a diagnosable condition, conventional medicine tends to be at a loss when faced with fatigue without a medical cause. Many doctors find themselves baffled when it comes to dealing with a person with long-standing fatigue that resists traditional medical tests. In fact, although there are many medical causes of tiredness, the great majority of tired people suffer from tiredness without a medical cause.

These days too, the doctor facing you over the surgery desk may be as tired as you are, if not more so! Doctors themselves can suffer from fatigue – in *How to Get the Best from Your Doctor* (Sheldon Press, 2007), Dr Tom Smith describes how earlier generations of doctors, constantly on call, died worn out in their 50s or 60s. Indeed, it's a sad fact that burn-out is increasing among medical professionals, among whom its prevalence has been estimated at more than 50 per cent. Possibly this is one reason why some doctors aren't always as sympathetic to their tired patients as they might be!

Communicating with your doctor

The classical patient–doctor relationship with regard to persistent tiredness is rather neatly summed up by the findings of a study published in the *British Medical Journal*, which showed that 61 per cent of patients perceived the cause of their tiredness to be physical, while 57 per cent of doctors viewed the problem as psychological. Generally, it seems that patients view tiredness as important because it affects their quality of life and can be disabling, whereas doctors do not, because by itself tiredness doesn't present specific enough grounds for diagnosis.

Obviously, this doesn't make for the ideal patient–doctor relationship. While doctors and health professionals are more informed about fatigue and fatigue syndromes than even a few years ago, the feedback from many people with severe sustained tiredness is that unhelpful attitudes are not yet extinct. Many people feel real anguish at not discovering a physical cause for their tiredness – especially if further investigation does unearth a cause.

> Nadine felt she had effectively lost two and a half years out of her life when she developed severe fatigue shortly after leaving university. 'Just as I should have been launching out into life, life suddenly closed in on me. I was permanently exhausted, found myself going to bed at 8p.m. every night and could barely hold down my job. My doctor prescribed antidepressants and when I refused to take them I felt I was labelled as a trouble-maker. In fact he told me quite clearly that my problem was psychiatric. I knew instinctively that it wasn't. I saw another doctor at the practice with similar results, after which I was too intimidated to go back for a year, during which time I soldiered on. Finally I went back and saw yet another doctor – luckily for me it was a large practice – who immediately asked if I'd been tested for thyroid disease. That was really the end of my nightmare. I was found to have an under-active thyroid and shortly afterwards I started medication. It was like picking up the pieces of my life from two and a half years before. I'm still angry that I wasn't taken seriously at first.'

Bear in mind that Nadine's story isn't typical – in most cases, no physical cause is ever found. In this kind of situation, though, it may help if you are meticulous about noting any other symptoms, in addition to your tiredness, and telling your doctor about these – even if you think they are minor. Symptoms that are regarded as medically significant are sometimes different from symptoms that you feel are causing you the most trouble, especially in disabling tiredness. However, because tiredness is so general, any other symptoms will give your doctor a clue as to possible underlying causes. For example, feeling the cold more and finding that your hair is limp and difficult to manage may be signs of a thyroid disorder – but you might well disregard such points in the face of your overwhelming tiredness. Think of your doctor and you as detectives together, and take all your symptoms seriously.

If this doesn't help, unless you have no choice of local GP, then you should seriously consider consulting another doctor if you can't get on with your present one and have been unable to resolve the difficulties by discussion. Unfortunately there is no national database of fatigue-friendly doctors! You do have the right to be referred to a specialist if you feel your GP is unable to help you as much as you would like. The waiting lists are unfortunately likely to be lengthy.

The medical approach to persistent tiredness

What conventional medicine can do is to test for a range of conditions that may underlie tiredness, such as anaemia, diabetes or heart trouble. Fatigue can be a symptom of, for example, an infection – a relatively short-lived one like flu, or a more prolonged one such as glandular fever or Lyme disease (also known as borrelia, an infection caused by the bite of a tick normally found on deer, and a condition that some increasingly believe is responsible for chronic fatigue). The fatigue of rheumatoid arthritis can be debilitating. Fatigue can be an early symptom of pregnancy, pre-menstrual syndrome, the perimenopause or the menopause – basically at any stage of a woman's reproductive life. It may accompany fibromyalgia, multiple sclerosis, undiagnosed urinary tract infection, anorexia or cancer; it may even foreshadow a heart attack. Medication may have fatigue as a side effect. One study of fatigue reported in the *British Medical Journal* breaks down possible medical causes of fatigue as follows:

- General – anaemia, chronic infection, autoimmune disease, cancer;
- Endocrine disease – diabetes, hypothyroidism, hypoadrenalism;
- Sleep disorders – obstructive sleep apnoea and other sleep disorders;
- Neuromuscular – myositis, multiple sclerosis;
- Gastrointestinal – liver disease;
- Cardiovascular – chronic heart disease;
- Respiratory – chronic lung disease.

Quite a choice. This isn't, of course, meant to worry you, but it does illustrate that persistent tiredness should always be checked out with your doctor to exclude the possibility of another condition; this is especially important if you have other symptoms such as swollen glands, weight loss, vomiting, shortness of breath, pain or soreness in the chest and abdomen.

However, even if persistent tiredness is your only symptom, it should always be taken seriously and checked out with your doctor. Fatigue is not something you should have to put up with – although sadly many people do.

The medical assessment

Stage one of any medical assessment is the taking of the person's history, combined with a clinical examination and preliminary medical investigations such as blood and urine tests. Depending on the nature of the symptoms or any findings discovered at this stage, the doctor will then explore further lines of enquiry as necessary.

Stage two of the medical assessment is to try to fit the history and findings with a satisfactory explanation. By 'satisfactory', doctors (and patients too) often mean a medical condition whose presence can be confirmed with a test, and probably treated with a drug or surgery – the hallmarks of Western medical treatment. The example of anaemia would be a typical such condition. It would be easily diagnosed with a blood sample, and if someone 'lacks blood' (the literal meaning of 'anaemia') to a sufficient degree then it would make complete sense that he or she should be fatigued as a result.

The results

Sometimes a specific cause for tiredness is found, such as an under-active thyroid gland, for which straightforward medical treatment may give complete relief. In most cases, though, as already stated, tiredness is not caused by an underlying illness.

It is much more usual to find that fatigue is a complicated problem for which a medical remedy is not obvious. In fact, a physical cause is found in only around 10 per cent of patients seeking help from their doctor. Our pattern of Western medical treatment often breaks down at this point. All the tests come back normal, and the results are that there is 'nothing wrong'.

Persistent tiredness usually has multiple causes

Tiredness can be caused by a number of factors working in combination, such as medical conditions, unhealthy lifestyle choices, workplace problems and stress. As stated in the Introduction, if one way to tackle tiredness already stood head and shoulders above the rest, then we'd all know about it – there's no dispute, for example, that insulin is the remedy for some types of diabetes. It's probably fair to say that there is no single best treatment because, often, fatigue is not just the result of one problem. This is where many existing 'remedies' for fatigue fail – they focus on single theories of why the tiredness is there in the first place. For example, people may blame their tiredness on food sensitivities or on lack of vitamins or on reactions to dental fillings, and, while strategies based on gluten-elimination diets or replacing old tooth fillings have worked for some, people who try these single-strategy treatments often end up being disappointed with the results.

Fatigue is often more complicated than this. If there is one statement that encapsulates the basic principles of fatigue recovery it is this: persistent tiredness usually has multiple causes. All the causes must be addressed before the tiredness will go away.

The good news is that people with persistent fatigue who have been thoroughly checked out by their doctor are unlikely to be suffering from a missed diagnosis of a very rare disease. That doesn't mean that all doctors diagnose correctable causes of tiredness first time. Nor is it to deny the acute frustration of people with chronic fatigue syndrome who are insulted by being persistently treated as psychiatric cases in the face of modern medicine's failure to find a physical cause for their condition. For the averagely tired person, however, it does mean that, once the doctor has given you a clean bill of health, you may have to do some work in terms of improving your sleep, diet and general lifestyle, which is where this book comes in.

Part of the problem is the tests themselves. We have perhaps rather got into the habit of expecting too much of modern medicine, and of thinking of tests as infallible. Modern medicine is often accused of a tendency towards over-reliance on technology. It's worth remembering, however, that many tests look for clinical results – that is, medically significant changes, not marginal ones that might make a difference to how you feel but aren't considered clinically significant. This may be one factor in why you sometimes emerge from the doctor's surgery with a clean bill of health, technically, but feeling just as awful as before. It would certainly appear that any abnormalities in chronic fatigue are subtle, because they do not show up on ordinary blood tests and the like – although that's not to say they aren't there. So, even with 'normal' results for blood tests, don't disregard persistent symptoms of fatigue, and don't give up. It may be that your body is sensitive to slight deficiencies that don't really need medication but that improve with better nutrition and rest. Have a look at Chapters 8 and 9.

A case in point – thyroid tests

It can be just as unhelpful for the doctor to find an abnormality in the tests that actually has little or nothing to do with someone's feeling of tiredness. For example, tests might reveal a slight abnormality of the thyroid gland – but, in practice, this may not be related to the fatigue the person is feeling; therefore, sometimes, even when attempts are made to correct the abnormality, the tiredness remains. In other words, medical tests aren't always the answer when it comes to finding the cause of tiredness, even when they do find something amiss! It should be noted, however, that treating thyroid dysfunction can have an impact on fatigue, as we'll see in Chapter 3.

Some causes of tiredness

As you can see from the information above, it's impossible to list all the possible medical causes of tiredness. Some of the most common, however, are outlined here, while thyroid disease is the subject of a short chapter after this one. Low blood sugar, a major physical cause of tiredness, is dealt with in Chapter 9, which looks at nutrition.

Anaemia

Iron-deficiency anaemia is the most common nutritional disorder in the world, affecting some 500 million people globally. As well as tiredness and weakness, other symptoms include shortness of breath after exertion, irritability, dizziness or fainting, palpitations, and pallor of the skin, lips, tongue, nail beds or the inside of eyelids.

Anaemia is an 'occupational hazard' if you are a woman of child-rearing age, especially if you have prolonged or heavy periods. Other causes of anaemia include internal bleeding, or a dietary deficiency of iron, folic acid or a failure to absorb vitamin B_{12} from the diet (pernicious anaemia). Anaemia may also be caused by chronic diseases like kidney disease, for example.

Your doctor can arrange a blood test for anaemia, and may prescribe iron. Some people prefer to take an organic supplement or tonic such as Floradix, available from pharmacies. Red meat and liver are good sources of iron, especially lamb and lamb's liver – generally, the darker the meat, the more iron it contains. Fish is also good, especially oily fish. Good sources of iron for vegetarians include wholegrain cereals and flours; leafy green vegetables, including spinach; blackstrap molasses; pulses, such as lentils and kidney beans; and some dried fruits, such as figs and apricots.

A diet that is very high in fibre may prevent the absorption of iron; tea or coffee drunk with a meal may have the same effect because they contain compounds called polyphenols, which inhibit absorption. Vitamin C, on the other hand, helps the body to absorb iron, which is why it's important to include sources of vitamin C, such as orange juice, fruit, vegetables or salads, in the diet.

Heart disease

While you shouldn't panic every time you get breathless or tired after exertion, it's worth remembering that coronary heart disease is the leading cause of death in the UK, killing around one in five men and one in six women. It is also the biggest single killer of women in the UK and USA.

Fatigue may be an early symptom of heart disease. You may feel tired most of the time, even when sitting or lying down. Even slight activity, such as making your bed, can result in overwhelming fatigue, which in this case is due to the reduced supply of oxygen to the muscles. Some women suffering from this just put it down to ageing.

There is some evidence to show that women may experience the symptoms of a heart attack differently from men. In a study of women who had heart attacks, unexplained fatigue or trouble sleeping were experienced as much as a month before the heart attack. The study at the University of Arkansas, led by Dr Jean C. McSweeney, was reported in *Circulation* (the journal of the American Heart Association). Other early warning symptoms noted in the study include shortness of breath, frequent indigestion and feelings of anxiety that come on for no known reason. Only about 30 per cent of women in the study mentioned the typical chest pain of heart attack as an early warning symptom, and when they did mention it they described the discomfort as an aching, pressure or burning rather than as a pain.

Heart failure also causes fatigue of the same overpowering nature. 'Failing' might be a better word than 'failure', because heart failure is an ongoing process whereby the heart loses its ability to pump blood effectively round the body. Other symptoms of heart failure include breathlessness, lack of energy, fluid retention and oedema (swelling) – especially of the ankles – and a general feeling of being unwell. Although heart failure affects both men and women, men are at slightly higher risk than women, reflecting the fact that heart attacks and angina, which can lead to heart failure, are slightly more common in men. Heart failure is estimated to affect around 900,000 people in the UK.

Medication, surgery and lifestyle changes can help with heart health, especially giving up smoking. In particular, brisk walking is also recommended – just 30 minutes a day five days a week.

Diabetes

Fatigue is a classic symptom of diabetes, one of the most under-diagnosed of medical conditions, so do see your doctor to rule this out, especially if you also tend to feel other symptoms such as increased thirst, a more frequent need to pass urine or blurred vision. A diagnosis can usually be made from a simple blood test. Type 1 diabetes is treated with diet and insulin injections; type 2 diabetes is treated more with lifestyle changes such as a healthier diet, weight loss and increased physical activity, as well as with drugs to lower blood glucose.

Insulin resistance

Insulin resistance is sometimes mentioned as a cause of fatigue. Insulin resistance occurs when normal amounts of insulin are produced by the body but there are problems with the body cells using it. Insulin resistance is one of the mechanisms by which diabetes happens. Weight loss can be very helpful – even a relatively small loss can have beneficial effects on blood glucose metabolism. Have a look at the advice on healthy eating in Chapter 9.

High blood pressure

Several studies have linked sleep apnoea, a sleep disorder that causes constant tiredness, with high blood pressure. For example, a study at the Johns Hopkins School of Public Health found that those who suffer from moderate to severe sleep apnoea were at increased risk of having high blood pressure. Another study found that more than 35 per cent of people with sleep apnoea suffer from high blood pressure, increasing their risk of heart disease.

Bear in mind that sleep apnoea is under-diagnosed; if you have the classic combination of snoring and daytime sleepiness, then it might be wise to consult your doctor. High blood pressure is usually symptomless, so if you haven't done so already, ask your GP or practice nurse for a check.

Low blood pressure

Low blood pressure is associated with fatigue, dizziness, weakness and depression. Not usually regarded as a serious health problem – generally, the lower the blood pressure, the lower the risk for stroke and heart disease – it can occasionally be a bit too much of a good thing. You probably know if you have low blood pressure but, if not, a home test can be getting up quickly after lying down and seeing if you feel dizzy (postural hypotension). Interestingly, yoga has been found useful for both low blood pressure and for chronic fatigue syndrome (see Chapter 12).

Polycystic ovary syndrome

Many women with polycystic ovary syndrome (PCOS) experience fatigue as a symptom as well as weight gain (despite their best efforts), irregular periods, acne and male-pattern hair growth. As PCOS is often linked to problems with insulin resistance, this could explain why tiredness is a common symptom.

In PCOS, the ovaries and sometimes the adrenal glands, for unknown reasons, pump out too much male hormone. Thinning hair, insulin resistance, excess facial hair, severe acne, irregular periods and impaired fertility are other symptoms to watch out for.

PCOS can be successfully managed with a low glycaemic diet and lifestyle changes. Some people may also be suitable for treatment with diabetes medication, especially if they're over-weight, which seems to reduce excess male hormones and to help to balance blood sugar levels.

'The tests are normal – you're fine'

So the doctor hasn't been able to help; maybe you've been dis-missed fairly briskly, or maybe with a few kindly, commonsense suggestions about getting more rest, cutting down a bit and asking others to help. Now what?

As we've said, these days we tend to expect a lot from medi-cine, especially as tests for illness become more subtle. However, the kinds of tests that your GP can do are enough to pick up most of the main detectable conditions that can cause fatigue. These kinds of tests will not pick up conditions such as chronic fatigue syndrome or psychological conditions such as depres-sion or anxiety, though GPs are skilled at detecting and treating these using other clinical skills.

If the test results are normal this does not mean the end of the story, nor should you feel crushed at 'having wasted the doc-tor's time' or feel as if you've been made to look a fool. Fatigue is a real condition that exists despite the absence of easily found abnormalities.

While over-estimating our ability to explain illness has rather left symptoms like tiredness out in the cold, it may be more helpful to forget the mind–body split for the time being. Once you have established that there is no apparent cause for your tiredness (such as diabetes, heart trouble or thyroid problems), it is far more useful to focus on ways of healing. Indeed, some research suggests that too intense a search for physical causes of tiredness can actually militate against getting better – as one study rather sourly put it, 'A preoccupation with medical causes seems to be a negative prognostic factor.'

Finally, as mentioned above, psychological factors may also be very important in fatigue, and these are discussed in Chapter 4. For more on chronic fatigue syndrome, see Chapter 12.

3

A word about the thyroid

A combination of fatigue and weight gain are two of the most common symptoms that bring people to see their family doctor. Although other causes of tiredness are more common – such as lack of sleep or depression – this combination can sometimes mean that the tiredness is due to changes in the way your thyroid works.

The thyroid is a little gland that controls your body's metabolic rate, or the speed at which the cells of your body work. If the human body were a car the thyroid gland would be the accelerator pedal. Its mechanism is in turn regulated by the master gland, the pituitary gland, situated in the 'third eye' position between the eyes.

The thyroid gland sits low in the front part of the neck, tucked away just below your Adam's apple, and produces a hormone that is released into the bloodstream and then distributed to all parts of the body. The hormone, called thyroxine, has an important role in the control of the body's use of energy – its metabolism. Mild disturbances of the thyroid gland, either under-activity or over-activity (usually the former) are relatively common. When the thyroid gland is markedly under-active, all sorts of problems occur. Apart from fatigue, there can be weight gain, swelling of the legs, sluggishness of muscles and speech, dry skin and hair, and a continuous feeling of being cold. Thyroxine is readily available as a tablet, and when given to someone who has very low thyroid activity the improvement can be quite remarkable.

Marked thyroid deficiency is, however, quite uncommon. Modern blood tests can detect very slightly low activity of the thyroid gland, the significance of which in terms of the person's symptoms may be highly debatable. So keen, though, are some doctors to find an 'organic' cause for their patient's tiredness that they will accept borderline low results as being significant. The tired person is told with confidence that the answer has been found, and that all they have to do is to take a little tablet of thyroxine every day. But when the person comes back for follow-up a few weeks later he or she feels just the same – the slightly low thyroid result has been a red herring.

In fairness it can be quite difficult to know in advance whether treatment with thyroxine will help someone whose tests suggest slight under-activity of the thyroid gland, in which case it must be tried out to see. But if the results are disappointing then one needs to look elsewhere for the causes of that person's fatigue. It is not uncommon to see in the medical notes of someone who has chronic fatigue the results of multiple thyroid tests, often done over quite short time spans, as one doctor after another prefers to search for an organic explanation, while in the meantime the patient isn't getting very much in the way of useful treatment.

Hypothyroidism

Hypothyroidism (under-active thyroid) is estimated to affect one in 50 women and one in 1,000 men. Because the thyroid hormone regulates the body's speed of activity, if levels of this hormone go down, your energy levels drop too; the whole of the body slows down, so needing less energy; this makes more energy available to be stored, leading to weight gain even if you actually feel less hungry. As well as causing tiredness and weight gain, hypothyroidism can result in other symptoms, including aches and pains, dry skin, lifeless hair and hair loss, feeling cold, and feeling sleepy and depressed. The general slowing down extends right to the intestines, making bowels slow and sluggish, and hence resulting in constipation.

Hyperthyroidism

Hyperthyroidism (overactive thyroid) represents a speeding up in the body's level of activity, so that more energy is used up and weight is lost; the raised levels of activity make the person feel warmer and make the brain work faster, sometimes resulting in irritability and insomnia. An increase in energy may seem to make tiredness unlikely but, paradoxically, sometimes the person may be too keyed up to sleep well, while the body can be worn out by symptoms such as shakiness, palpitations, rapid pulse and diarrhoea, resulting in a drop in overall energy, fatigue, and feelings of weakness and lethargy.

Thyroid hormones

A complicating factor in thyroid gland under-activity concerns the exact nature of the medication used to treat it. To go into full details on this topic would be too much of a diversion into biochemistry, but a brief summary is justified because it is a controversial topic upon which some people with chronic fatigue have strong views – especially if they have found themselves helped by the treatment deemed controversial!

The molecule that is called thyroxine is fairly uncomplicated to a chemist and is quite easily synthesized. Essential ingredients of thyroxine are atoms of iodine (which is why dietary iodine deficiency, rarely seen in the UK, can cause under-activity of the thyroid gland). Thyroxine contains four atoms of iodine; hence it is often referred to in shorthand as T4.

Thyroxine exerts its influence on the cells of the body by causing changes to the DNA of the cells. It does this by moving in from the bloodstream to within the cell nucleus, where the DNA is located. Before becoming attached to the DNA, however, one atom of iodine is removed, producing T3. T3 is therefore thought to be the active form of thyroid hormone, rather than T4.

T4 is, however, the molecule that is the most commonly used as treatment for people who need extra thyroid hormone. It lasts longer than T3, needing only one dose a day, whereas T3 is short-lived and needs to be given two or three times per day. According to the vast majority of thyroid experts around the world, the process by which the body makes T3 from T4 is almost never faulty. There should therefore be little or no need for anyone to take T3 in preference to T4.

Many people with an under-active thyroid gland who do not feel much better on standard thyroxine treatment disagree. They have found that treatment with T3 does them more good. Other people go further and feel better only by taking an extract made from the dried thyroid glands of pigs, thereby avoiding synthetic thyroxine completely.

It's not the intention of this section to take sides in this debate, but it does raise some important matters that are relevant to chronic fatigue.

Some people say that they feel better with thyroid hormone treatment

Despite the expert opinion saying that it should not matter, there are plenty of people who are adamant that it does. Who is right? Surely the person's experience is what matters?

Some patients say that thyroid hormone treatment makes no difference

If someone has a problem other than reduced thyroid gland activity that's keeping him or her back, treating only the thyroid gland will not bring about a cure.

Maybe there is too much 'science' going on

Some people can undoubtedly become a bit too fixed on the idea that if only they could tweak the thyroid hormones a bit more to suit their individual needs, they'd feel a lot better. Although this might be correct for some people, for others it might be a distraction that prevents them looking elsewhere for more relevant reasons to explain their fatigue. It's an understandable part of the search for a definable cause and cure.

The truth is that while abnormal activity of the thyroid gland, then, is a 'diagnosable' cause of chronic fatigue, borderline low blood test results may be misleading and not truly the cause of a person's fatigue.

Too much more on the thyroid is really beyond the scope of this book, but the support organization Thyroid UK has an excellent, informative website at <http://www.thyroiduk.org/>.

Yoga for the thyroid

Because medication is not always the definitive answer to thyroid problems, some people may be interested to know that yogis traditionally recommend certain yoga postures to help.

Two of the postures recommended are the shoulder stand (sarvangasana) and the plough. You can find these poses demonstrated on the internet, which may be a good way to start – although ideally you should find a gentle yoga class (no power yoga until you feel a bit more energized) so you can ensure that you are practising the poses correctly. Read right to the end before you try it as you should warm up first.

Warm-up exercises

If you are not a yoga devotee, do not try to do the shoulder stand or the plough straight off – and even if you are, you should warm up first. Warm-up yoga exercises and poses can be found on the internet (for example, see <http://www.will-harris. com/yoga>), and some sites show the actual movements that need to be made.

Some warm-ups might include:

• Rocking – lie on your back, with your hands tucked beneath your knees, and the knees brought into your chest; rock to and fro 10 times.

- Stretching – stand tall with your fingers interlaced, your palms facing outwards; keeping your legs straight, breathe out and stretch to the right; hold for a few moments, breathing freely; inhale, and repeat to the left as you exhale.

The shoulder stand

Space out the steps to the shoulder stand gradually over a few days if you are not accustomed to yoga, or when working up to a shoulder stand in the morning.

To perform the shoulder stand, do the following steps.

1 Lie on your back and raise your legs a few inches in the air. Keep your legs straight.
2 Still lying on your back, bring your legs right up so that you form an L-shape with torso and legs.
3 Now bring your legs backwards towards your shoulders.
4 Tuck your hands beneath the small of your back and raise yourself gradually.
5 Finally, raise yourself right up on to your shoulders, or as far as you can go.

Wonderfully energizing!

The plough

To perform the plough, do the following steps.

1 Bring your knees rapidly into your chest, raising up your pelvis and lower back. Straighten your legs when the lower back begins to rise.
2 Take the legs slowly down behind your head and place your hands into the lower back for support.
3 If possible allow the legs to come all the way down to the mat.

4

All in your head? Emotions, depression and anxiety

Few things are more infuriating than having someone suggest that your tiredness is all in your head, especially if you have been to the doctors and come back with a clean bill of health. The 'snap out of it' school may be particularly inappropriate if you have depression or anxiety, which are the main subjects of this chapter. First, though, a word about something that causes a lot of confusion – the role of the emotions in illness. Some people have had the distressing experience of being sent away from the doctor's with no diagnosis only to find on a return visit – sometimes years later – that they do have a physical condition such as thyroid trouble or diabetes. Others have found themselves landed with a most unwelcome and inappropriate psychiatric diagnosis.

One school of thought, however, says that emotions, especially emotions from our earlier years, can become 'encoded' in the body, dictating later patterns of health.

Your biography, your biology?

'I can't stomach it any longer,' 'It's a pain in the neck' and, perhaps most relevantly for this book, 'I'm sick and tired of it.' We constantly use illness metaphors to express how we're feeling. But can our emotions really make us physically ill?

This is obviously a simplification of what promises to be a complex biochemical process. Simplistically, then, we do know that, for example:

- stress can disrupt the body's hormonal balance, leading to symptoms (see Chapter 6); and
- depression and anxiety may have physical symptoms.

The traditional allopathic view of conventional medicine says that health is a matter of genes, exposure to infection and lifestyle. Western medicine has a bad name for ignoring the emotional components of illness. However, some research has shown a correlation between earlier emotional experience and certain conditions, such as heart disease, depression and chronic pain, and suggests that some illness is emotions that have been biologized. The ACE study, run by the Centers for Disease Control and Prevention in the USA, assesses the link between emotional experience in earlier life (adverse childhood events, or ACE) and adult health in more than 17,000 people. Results to date show that those who have experienced an adverse childhood event such as neglect or trauma were between four and 50 times more likely to have an adverse health condition or disease as an adult, including heart disease, fractures, diabetes, obesity and alcoholism. It's easy to understand this on a behavioural basis – that is, our past experiences may direct us to make unhealthy choices such as smoking or drinking too much – but whether such events have any actual biological effect needs more research.

For practical purposes, two conclusions stand out when considering fatigue.

- The traditional mind–body split may not be the most helpful way of approaching tiredness. While the more traditional allopathic viewpoint focuses more on 'physical' and 'psychological' illnesses as being separate, to a certain extent both elements are involved in all illnesses.
- Once your doctor has established there is no obvious cause for your tiredness, including depression (see below), it is usually more useful to focus on healing than to continue to hunt for a cause, despite the very natural 'need to know';

many mechanisms of healing are independent of the cause of the illness.

Boredom

As well as doing too much, boredom can be a prime factor in tiredness, as Janine found.

Janine had been a keen athlete at school and university, and still enjoyed physical fitness. When left at home with two small children, however, she became exhausted – so much so that she would have to lie down every day between 4p.m. and 6p.m., when her husband came home. She then started going out to work two days a week, and to the gym three times every week. The effect was magical; what had been over-powering fatigue, strong enough to fell her for the day, mysteriously vanished within 15 minutes once she got out of the house. Of course the exercise revived her, but the effect started well before she even reached the gym, and she felt the same when on the way to work, where she received stimulus and company. Although she adored her children, being alone with them all week was too much of a good thing. Her tiredness was boredom.

Pacing yourself and avoiding over-activity

Obvious though it may be, the need to pace themselves can often be overlooked by tired people, especially if they've previously been able to take their energy for granted.

The temptation is, when you feel strong and energetic, to run round catching up with everything and trying to do what you think ought to be done in a full day. The key is to pace yourself, and to hold some energy in reserve, rather than squandering it all when you do feel well. Often a tired person is a 'coper' – someone who typically lives life (or two or three lives) to the full – working, caring, shopping, cleaning – and only ever resting when asleep, until the tiredness strikes. As Trudie Chalder explains in her book *Coping with Chronic Fatigue* (Sheldon Press, 2002), planned rest – preferably at the same time or times every day – is much more effective than resting because you have to – that is, when you drop from sheer exhaustion. So, it's best to plan rest times into your day, and rest before you are tired, at the same time or times every day – perhaps mid-morning and mid-afternoon if practicable – and not to wait until you are tired. Keep a daily record of how much you do and how much physical activity you have, and see if you can pace yourself so that you have roughly the same amount of *manageable* activity every day, with rests in between. Spread tasks out so that you don't, for example, spend every Wednesday or Saturday working, shopping or cleaning from dawn until dusk – if necessary, spread one day's work over three days.

Is tiredness dissatisfaction?

Alice was a passionate art student and was thrilled when she got a place in a Saturday class at a London academy. At first, she came home on fire with it all, making copious notes on the train on the way back. After four years, however, she found it increasingly hard to go – she overslept every Saturday morning, was sleepy in class and fell asleep on the train coming back. She had outgrown the class, and shortly afterwards gave it up, moving on.

Is tiredness an escape?

Tiredness can sometimes prevent people engaging with the very problems that make them tired.

June had an unhappy marriage but hated confrontation and dreaded being lonely; Jodie hated where she lived but couldn't face the problem of moving; Peter disliked his well-paid job and wanted to move on. All were, however, too tired on a daily basis to start making the necessary small changes that would have moved them on. The 'pay-off' of tiredness was that it allowed them not to deal with underlying life problems. The mental fatigue of being stuck added to their burden of tiredness.

Depression

Depression is one of the most common conditions to afflict human beings. Some 5–10 per cent of the population have some degree of depression over the course of a year – but it's often a hidden condition. Depression, and mental illness in general, are conditions we don't like to talk about much, or admit to having. Unfortunately, the stigma that accompanies depression often makes people feel a 'failure' or as if they are 'weak' when depression strikes. But depression, as well as being common, is also highly treatable, and treatment does not always have to be with antidepressant drugs. It can be enough just to have depression acknowledged and discussed.

Depression is a bit of a medical chameleon – it can take many forms. It often appears as a physical illness first, such as fatigue, which is one reason why so many doctors like to pounce on it as a possible 'bucket diagnosis'. Chronic illness, and persistent fatigue, can also precipitate depression for the first time.

Symptoms

There are many recognized symptoms of depression, which don't always occur at the same time:

- low mood;
- inability to gain pleasure from activities that are normally pleasurable;
- loss of interest in normal activities, hobbies and everyday life;
- feeling tired all the time and having no energy;
- difficulty getting off to sleep, or waking up early in the morning;
- feeling unable to get out of bed and 'face the world';
- loss of appetite and interest in food;
- weight change – either a loss in weight due to decreased appetite or an increase in weight from 'comfort eating';
- loss of interest in sex;
- difficulty in concentration, as in trouble reading or being able to 'think straight';
- feeling restless, tense or anxious;
- being irritable;
- losing self-confidence;

- avoiding other people;
- finding it harder than usual to make decisions;
- feeling useless and inadequate – 'a waste of space';
- feeling guilty about who you are and what you have done;
- feeling hopeless – that nothing will make things better;
- thinking about suicide.

Some of these symptoms, such as fatigue, irritability, appetite disturbance and so on have been experienced by virtually everyone at some point in their lives. Other symptoms – especially suicidal ideas, marked hopelessness or guilt – are outside the normal range of mood. When those are present the diagnosis of depression might be all too obvious, but it is much more common to have the less dramatic symptoms.

Often depression is quite obvious to the sufferer and to his or her family, friends and workmates; however, other people are quite good at hiding their depression, or it may come across as irritability or a general impression that someone's personality has changed.

Seasonal affective disorder

Tiredness is a recognized part of seasonal affective disorder (SAD) or winter depression. Many people in northern climes feel low in the winter or go into a type of hibernation mode, with minor changes in energy, appetite, mood and sleep. One in 20, however, suffers from SAD, in which a lack of natural daylight causes changes in energy, appetite, mood and sleep patterns that are significant enough to interfere with normal living. SAD is marked by fatigue and over-sleeping, craving for carbohydrates and corresponding weight gain, social isolation and withdrawal from people, and depression.

The growth of SAD may be due in part to our indoor 21st-century lifestyle, as we spend at least three-quarters of daily life under artificial light, whereas, in pre-electricity days, work was geared towards daylight, taking place either outside or near to windows during daylight. While lack of daylight is most likely in winter, other times we may not get enough natural light could be, for example, when working long hours indoors or when working at night. Wearing glasses may also screen out natural daylight.

The cause of SAD isn't really known, but one theory is that we simply don't get enough natural light on our eyes, which acts as a wake-up call to the body. This is especially true in the morning, when light hitting the eyes signals to the brain, more specifically the pineal gland, to stop producing melatonin, the substance that makes us drowsy at night. Melatonin production is linked with our circadian rhythm, the process that helps regulate our internal body clock, and tells us when to sleep and when to wake up. Disruption of this natural body clock may cause depression. Exposure to bright lights has also been linked with the production of serotonin, lack of which causes depression.

SAD does need to be differentiated from clinical depression or manic depression (bipolar disorder), which can also have cycles throughout the year.

Light therapy is a standard as well as the obvious treatment for SAD. Some people find more exposure to daylight helpful; others find they don't benefit unless they have access to a device that emits really bright light. This might mean, for example, having a bright lamp at the breakfast table, wearing a cap with a special light for an hour in the morning or having an alarm clock (dawn simulator) that uses gradually increasing light as a wake-up device (see Useful addresses).

There is some evidence to show that light therapy may help those with chronic fatigue syndrome. One study showed that more than a third of people with chronic fatigue syndrome found their symptoms were worse in winter; in fact, over-sleeping, daytime fatigue, carbohydrate craving and eating were indistinguishable from these same features in people with SAD. Research at Columbia University Medical Center, New York, and the and University of British Columbia, Vancouver, showed marked improvement in people using light therapy, not just in SAD-like symptoms such as daytime tiredness, but also in physical symptoms of chronic fatigue syndrome (such as joint pain) that are rarely seen in SAD. Light therapy may also be helpful for people who fall asleep too early or who can't go to sleep until late and then oversleep in the morning, because bright light is believed to help reset the body clock. Some research has also found it helpful with pre-menstrual syndrome – both for psychological and physical symptoms.

Dealing with depression

If you suspect you have depression, do go and see your doctor. Depression is very treatable. Non-drug treatments can be effective for depression, such as counselling, cognitive behavioural therapy (CBT) or other types of 'talking treatment' – the UK government has pledged to spend £170 million on 'talking treatments' over the next decade. Modern antidepressant drug treatment often works very well and is safe, although it meets with different responses in different people and doesn't suit everyone; some people experience side effects, and some find psychological treatments as effective as drug treatment, if not more so.

Anxiety

Anxiety often accompanies depression, and may be the more important component of someone's illness. Some degree of anxiety is quite normal, for example at a job interview. Being anxious about flying or crossing a busy street heightens our awareness of the risks involved, and so can be seen as a realistic help to us in everyday life. When anxiety becomes a problem, or an illness, it is because it lasts too long, or the symptoms are more severe, or they impair our ability to function in physical ways or in social or occupational situations.

Anxiety is common – taken over a lifetime about 30 per cent of people probably suffer from it. Mixed anxiety and depression is present in about 11 per cent of women and 7 per cent of men at any one time.

Symptoms

The symptoms of anxiety can be thought of in two groups – those affecting the body and those affecting the mind. Some of each are always present in an affected person.

Physical symptoms of anxiety include:

- sweating;
- fast pulse and palpitations;
- dry mouth and difficulty swallowing;
- shaking of muscles (tremor);
- chest tightness or breathlessness;
- numbness or tingling of the fingers and toes and around the mouth (caused by hyperventilation – see below);
- feeling faint;
- increased frequency of passing urine;
- diarrhoea;
- hyperventilation syndrome (multiple symptoms such as pins and needles of the hands and a feeling of faintness brought on by breathing too quickly).

Psychological symptoms of anxiety include:

- fear and apprehension;
- irritability;
- inner tension;
- poor concentration;
- increased sensitivity to being startled or to physical sensations;
- disturbed sleep;
- worries about losing control or losing your mind;
- worries about being sick, fainting or having a heart attack.

5

The rhythm of life: being too busy

One simple cause of tiredness that is often ignored, especially by multi-tasking women, is doing too much – cramming more into a day than would have been dreamed of even a couple of generations ago. The old English nursery rhyme set this out clearly:

Wash on Monday,
Iron on Tuesday,
Mend on Wednesday,
Churn on Thursday,
Clean on Friday,
Bake on Saturday,
Rest on Sunday.

The English tradition of washing clothes on a Monday was taken to America when the women of the Mayflower came ashore on Monday 13 November 1620 and the first thing they did – typically – was the washing, thus perpetuating the great tradition of busy, working, tired women.

This is not to advocate a return to old times past for the sake of nostalgia, nor a call to romantic slowing down for its own sake – would you really want to go back to washing say 40 or more soiled cloth nappies, the entire family's sheets and towels, and all the clothes, by hand every Monday? It does underline, however, the point that only one major activity was expected to be done a day.

Today, technological advances allow us to get so much more done that the pace of life has literally speeded up; we are harangued by technology. This is illustrated, perhaps tongue in cheek, by a much-publicized walking survey in 32 cities, which revealed that average walking speeds have increased by about 10 per cent since 1994. The findings apparently reflect the way that technology such as the internet and mobile phones have made people more impatient, leading them to cram more and more activities into a day. Richard Wiseman, a professor of psychology at the University of Hertfordshire, who led the study, said that the results were significant because walking speed was a good indicator of the pace of people's lives. The danger is that as people get more stressed and hurried, they spend less time relaxing with friends, exercising or eating properly, and they tend to drink and smoke more.

Previous research by Robert Levine, of California State University, who measured walking speeds around the world in 1994, showed that they are linked to other indicators of behaviour and health. As people move faster they become less likely to help others, and they tend to have higher rates of coronary heart disease.

Measuring your pace

To measure your pace Wiseman (author of *Quirkology*, PanMacMillan) has devised the following test. He says that if you have five or more 'yes' answers, then you may want to slow down.

1 Do you seem to glance at your watch more than others?
2 When someone takes too long to get to the point, do you want to hurry them along?
3 Are you often first to finish at meal times?
4 When walking along a street, do you feel frustrated because you are stuck behind others?
6 Would you become irritable if you sat for an hour with nothing to do?
7 Do you walk out of restaurants or shops if you encounter a short queue?
8 If you are caught in slow-moving traffic, do you seem to get more annoyed than other drivers?

As noted above, five or more 'yes' responses means that you should take your foot off the accelerator.

Others, however, say that spending less time on inessential activities such as walking allows you to spend more time on what really matters. Anna Travis, for example, writing at the news commentary e-zine *spiked* – <http://www.spiked-online.com/index.php?/site/> – calls a halt to the cult of slowness for its own sake, which is often snobbery and elitism in disguise, as well as a withdrawal from life! The key is discrimination in how we choose to spend our time, something that can be steam-rollered by our cram-it-in society. The pseudo-allure of being busy can become glamorized in a consumer culture where time is another commodity.

Being busy, then, is probably one of the most common causes of tiredness, especially among women. If you can't resist the temptation to be all things to all people, it's worth calling a halt to everything and asking yourself just why. Is it really demanded – or even expected – of you? Could it just be habit? What are you staying so busy for? Is there anything you can let go of?

According to the dictionary, busy means 'engaged in action'. However, it is also defined as overcrowded or cluttered with detail – 'a busy painting', 'a fussy design' – as well as inter-fering – 'busy about other people's business'.

'Busy' is the standard response when people ask each other how they are, often said with a simpering self-consciousness that implies they are the only ones suffering this affliction. Indeed, because we're all busy, busy is a meaningless word.

Being busy is often essentially counterproductive and can mean that you're not in control, that tasks are working them-selves through you in an never-ending line with ever-diminishing time. Activities you previously enjoyed may become drudgery as task after task is ticked off in the ceaseless battle to 'get it all done'. This isn't to advocate a mindless slowing down for its own sake. It's about choice, not pace – doing what feels right to you, not to someone else. Tiredness is often a message that life is full to overflowing, although not necessarily with what you really want to be doing. Pay attention! Because if you don't make some conscious choices about what needs to go, there is the risk that your body will shout louder and louder, with more intense fatigue, so forcing you to call a halt anyway.

> Hannah, like many fatigued people, had always been busy but found that, although her days were as packed as ever, she seemed to be getting less and less done. Tasks that were routine a few months ago became difficult chores, and her pace seemed to become slower and slower. She noticed this particularly in shopping – previously something that she tucked into an evening after work now took up a whole morning; not only was she much slower getting round the supermarket, but she also needed to rest afterwards after the gruelling task of unloading it all and putting it away. Shopping was the tip of the iceberg – just one task too many in her busy life.

How busy are you?

To see how busy you are, try writing down your routine for a single day, including activities such as preparing clothes for work or school in the morning, taking children to school, commuting, caring for any pets, shopping, preparing meals, work, socializing, attendance at any committees, voluntary activities, school or work involvements, and assorted tasks such as family or friends' birthdays, picking up dry-cleaning, taking books back to the library and so on.

Surprised? Now, use a daily journal for two weeks to identify causes of fatigue or things that make you overtired as opposed to just tired (for example, staying late at work, going to bed half an hour too late, talking on the phone in the evening when tired and so on).

Now, ask yourself these questions.

- Why am I so busy, and for whom – myself, my family, my parents (even if deceased), my work?
- What, if anything, am I postponing by being so busy? Is 'busy-ness' distracting me from an unsatisfactory lifestyle or poor performance at work?
- Is being busy 'interfering' with anything (that is, with what I feel I really want to be doing)?
- How could I do less and achieve more?
- Is being busy easier than calling a halt and paying attention to the parts of my life that really need it?

- Am I busy packing in the unessential? Or am I hanging on to tasks that it's really time to pass on to someone else?
- How could it benefit me – and others – if I stopped being so busy?
- Do I know the difference between a busy day and a fully lived day?
- Is my tiredness telling me something about aspects of my lifestyle that I dislike or that I've outgrown?
- Is my tiredness forcing me to stop being busy?

A daily 'stop-doing' list

The brilliant idea of having a daily 'stop-doing' list is suggested by Jim Collins in *Good to Great* (HarperCollins, 2001). He makes the distinction between a disciplined life and a busy life. Being busy is all about making choices – or rather, not making choices; in other words, being busy and overstretched is a natural result of not making clear choices about priorities.

It may help to imagine having choices forced upon you. Jim Collins suggests that you imagine you receive two phone calls – the first telling you that you have inherited $20 million, no strings attached, the second that you have an incurable terminal disease, with no more than 10 years to live. What would you do differently, and, in particular, what would you stop doing?

Especially when we're tired and so can't do everything we'd like to anyway, how we best choose to spend our precious energy becomes an even more vital question. In other words, which one, two or more activities can we drop? How do we prioritize?

Jim Collins suggests three key questions.

1 What are you deeply passionate about?
2 What are you are genetically encoded for – what activities do you feel just 'made to do'?
3 What makes economic sense – what can you make a living at?

Collins also points out that, when you decide what to do, sometimes something is inevitably lost. It means saying 'no'. It means admitting, perhaps painfully or uncomfortably, that we can't do everything. This may mean saying goodbye to projects in which we may already have substantially invested, in terms of time and effort, but doing what you really want to do means being focused and self-disciplined. However, he adds, it is this discipline 'that distinguishes the truly exceptional artist and marks the ideal piece of work, be it a symphony, a novel, a painting, a company or, most important of all, a life.'

This obviously applies not just to those who are tired – Collins writes primarily in a business context – but to those who need to make life decisions, which is all of us.

So, for example, Hannah's 'stop-doing' list looked like this.

- Stop answering email immediately it arrives – save it all up for a session at the end of the morning or day.
- Stop seeing people who exhaust me. Most meetings with people take an hour to an hour and a half, but that's enough to wipe out my energy for the morning or even the day.
- Stop answering the phone or mobile.
- Stop shopping and let my partner do it!
- Stop starting the day with routine tasks like washing up – do the important things first when I'm fresh, then save up housework and so on for the afternoon.
- Stop visiting my mother-in-law so often – it's an awful, exhausting drive of 50 minutes through heavy traffic and I get nothing out of it beyond the feeling that I've done my duty.

Planned rest

It's natural to wait until we're tired and then rest. In particular, many women's pattern is to rush around until they drop. How many times have you said, any time from the early evening onwards, 'I'm fine so long as I don't sit down'? Collapsing into a chair, say at 6p.m. or onwards, signals the end of the day and the steady slide towards bedtime! Planning rest into your day, however, aims at conserving that precious energy and preventing tiredness. The secret is to pace yourself.

- As far as possible, plan rest into your day, as much as possible at around the same time each day – say two periods of 30–45 minutes in the morning and afternoon, or an hour and a half in the middle of the day.
- This rest time should be yours absolutely, without distractions, in which to read, think or listen to music.
- Don't sleep, unless you have no sleeping problems and know that a brief nap suits you and restores your energy.
- If you do feel sleepy, try going to bed half an hour or an hour earlier.
- Avoid doing too much when you feel energetic – this tends to lead to burn-out and exhaustion later on the same day, or the following day.
- 'I don't have time to rest.' You're doing too much! Have a look at your timetable and see where you could cut down to make time to rest.
- 'I get bored resting.' Audio CDs cover a wide range of subjects, so why not occupy your mind by learning a foreign language or new business; craftwork or artwork are also options, such as rug making, working with doll's houses or accessories, making model boats or knitting.

How to say 'no'

Saying 'no' can be painful or uncomfortable; and, for tired people, it can take energy! There is a saying, however, that if it's right for you, it's right for others – certainly, it's rare that people will be as hurt or inconvenienced as you might imagine if you do refuse a task or an invitation. How often do you say 'yes' to please others or because you simply don't have your priorities – that is, your life – clear enough in your mind?

Prioritize! Make a list of everything that you have to do, feel you need to do or think you should do. Accept the fact that when you were healthy you may have been able to handle everything, but that now some things are going to have to change if you are going to have any quality of life. Evaluate every item on your list by asking yourself how important and necessary this is and whether someone else can help or do this for you. Also consider whether you are doing this because you want to or because someone else thinks you should. The only items that should remain on your list are those that are truly important to you or are a necessity.

The fact that we have limited time, and limited energy, takes on more significance in times of tiredness. Indeed, fatigue's most vital message might be to tell us that we can't do everything, and that sometimes saying 'no' to some things is the best way of saying 'yes' to what really matters to us in life.

Finally, choosing to be busy doesn't in itself cause stress; many people thrive on it. However, feeling that we have an overly busy lifestyle imposed from the outside can be stressful. For more on tackling stress, read on to the next chapter.

6

Stress and stress hormones

Feeling powerless is a large part of both stress and of feeling tired, and stress is a recognized trigger factor for fatigue to develop and continue – it's a noted 'block to recovery'.

We tend to put ourselves through stresses and strains on a daily basis, usually without much immediate thought for the consequences. By the time stress has us in its grip, we often feel it's too late to exercise our power – we're entangled. However, making even simple choices and decisions can help us break free.

Serious attention should be paid to the matters that are giving rise to the most worry and put them into one of two categories:

- those you can do nothing about; and
- those that can be reduced with the right action.

If your worries are in the first category, do try and detach from them as much as you can. This doesn't mean you have to avoid thinking about them, but if you genuinely have no control over their outcome, it's okay to tuck them to one corner of your mind, get your hot water bottle and go to bed.

Regarding the second category, make a list and choose something to tackle. Ideally, it should be the most important point, and only when that is done should you tackle another. However, some people find it helpful to start with a relatively trivial task such as washing up or buying new socks – anything that makes us feel, however humbly, back in control.

Another good way to feel back in control is to have a spring-clean, even on a small scale – such as a drawer, your desk or your car. Clutter creates confusion and can be tiring as well.

Relaxation is something we should all be doing anyway – if only we had the time! Take more time for yourself – it's a very effective way of helping yourself to recover. Forget about bombing around, or that you lack the ability at present to do so, and instead step into a more relaxed mode. The world will rotate at exactly the same speed either way. Yoga, meditation, massage and aromatherapy are popular for good reasons and they can encourage you to discover the lost art of relaxation. Perhaps you used to have a hobby that you enjoyed but that got sidelined by a lack of time, or perhaps there is some other pastime that you haven't previously tried but that takes your fancy. It need not be expensive – most of the investment is your time.

Many aspects of modern life are incredibly stressful, and if the stressful situation can't be changed, what we need to do is change the way we respond to stress. Try to think of stress in a more positive light. Stress is the spice of life. In the words of Hans Selye, the doctor who conducted early research into the effects of stress on the body, 'Complete freedom from stress is death because all human activity involves stress.'

Our bodies can't distinguish between what is real stress or emergency and what isn't. Many of the things we get worked up about aren't really so very important.

Dealing with stress: a three-point plan

Often, part of stress is feeling caught up in a situation that is too complex to remedy. So, keep it simple. If you do only the three things on this list you will have made significant progress towards de-stressing your life.

1 *Identify stress triggers.* What causes you stress? Work pressures? A family situation? Poor housing? Commuting? Don't over-look the small but significant ones.
2 *Get a good night's sleep.* This is one of the simplest and easiest

ways to cope with stress. Defy the sleep experts and have a lie-in, too (see Chapter 3).
3 *Get more time to yourself.* Beg, borrow or steal this – even if it's just five minutes here and there. Will anyone really notice if you have a 20-minute break? A 30-minute one? A whole hour, afternoon or day to yourself? Why not try it and see?

Stress hormones

One reason why stress is tiring is because it floods the body with stress hormones such as cortisol and adrenaline – which are good in small doses – far in excess of need. These hormones are manufactured by the all-important adrenal glands, which sit on top of the kidneys just under the last rib. They are controlled by other hormones circulating in the bloodstream, which come originally from the pituitary gland of the brain, which in turn is controlled by the hypothalamus – the central control centre of the brain. The adrenal glands secrete more than 50 hormones that play vital roles in the body, including the 'stress hormones' adrenaline and cortisol. In addition, the adrenal glands are responsible for many of the functions essential to health, such as converting carbohydrate, protein and fat to blood glucose for energy; balancing fluids and electrolytes in the body; and fat storage.

Cortisol in particular plays an important role in keeping the body in balance. It helps to regulate blood pressure and blood sugar, and balances the immune system.

Adrenal exhaustion

These functions go awry in adrenal exhaustion, a process that tends to happen over a period of time. The adrenal glands are designed to react quickly, like a gun going off in self-defence, not continuously. What often happens when we're under stress is that we subject the adrenal glands to repeated attacks until they start losing the ability to 'fire'.

When you are faced with a stressful situation, your adrenal glands start to release cortisol, the 'fight or flight' hormone; just in case you do need to fight or run away fast. Cortisol increases the fat and sugar in your bloodstream that your brain and muscles use for a quick burst of energy. So, in times of stress, cortisol may be released at about 20 times its normal rate. After the anxiety has passed, your body returns to its normal state.

Unfortunately, today, the stress response is usually inappropriate; a surge in stress hormones is of no use to us when we're stuck on a crowded tube or at a desk trying to sort out an intractable work problem. Surges in stress hormones are fine now and again, but sustained high levels of stress hormones can have a damaging effect on your heart, stomach, hormonal balance and psychological health, weakening the immune system and slowing down healing. For example, the blood supply decreases to the digestive system, and having a digestive system on constant shut down certainly militates against getting the most out of your nutrition.

In adrenal exhaustion, the adrenal glands, which do the work of releasing cortisol, become exhausted by the constant demands of stress, and are able to release less and less cortisol. Tiredness takes on particular characteristics in adrenal fatigue. You may find that:

- you're especially tired in the morning and can't seem to get going until you've been awake for a couple of hours;
- you suffer mid-afternoon dips – low energy and fuzzy thinking from 2p.m. to 4p.m.;
- you may have an early evening revival around 6p.m., with higher energy then; and
- you may have another second wind later in the evening after 10p.m.

As well as tiredness, adrenal fatigue symptoms include feeling that:

- you've lost the ability to bounce back from stress;
- you have allergies, inflammation or digestive problems;
- you can't lose excess weight even when trying to;
- you need caffeine or carbohydrates as boosters;
- you crave salty, sugary or fatty foods; and
- pre-menstrual syndrome worsens.

Normally, cortisol levels are highest in the morning, when you get up, and then decline gradually until they reach the lowest levels at bedtime. What often seems to happen in severe, sustained adrenal fatigue is that this pattern is reversed, leaving you keyed up and over-stimulated at night, unable to wind down enough to sleep. This helps to explain why some tired people get a second wind at night, or fall fast asleep early, only to wake up at 2a.m. or 3a.m. unable to go back to sleep, minds racing.

How to deal with adrenal exhaustion

To help to break the vicious cycle, minimize stress and negativity – follow the suggestions for relaxing and cutting down on stress (see above). A healthy diet will help – follow the advice in Chapter 9. In particular, avoid junk food; cut down on carbohydrates, caffeine and alcohol; and include essential fatty acids and lots of vegetables – six small servings a day if you can. Ensure your food is rich in calcium, magnesium, vitamin C, vitamin E and vitamin B complex. It may be worth taking a multi-vitamin and mineral supplement for a while.

The adrenal glands not only produce cortisol but a range of other hormones. One is dehydroepiandrosterone (DHEA), which helps to govern the balance of hormones in the body and is a precursor hormone to oestrogen, progesterone and testosterone. When the adrenal glands don't produce enough DHEA, as can happen if they are struggling with large amounts of cortisol, symptoms can include tiredness, depression, aching joints and decreased sex drive. As you'll see in the next chapter, the sex hormones play quite a part in fatigue.

7

Hormonal factors for women: pre-menstrual syndrome, pregnancy, menopause

In general, women are twice as likely as men to have difficulties falling or staying asleep, with problems being more common in women over 40. Tiredness in women is often put down to hormonal factors, which seem to affect women at any stage of reproductive life you care to mention. Some women feel more tired at certain times of the month than at others. Others get to know exhaustion along with pregnancy, birth and a new baby. Again, some women start feeling more tired than usual in the run up to menopause.

Menstruation

Hormonal fluctuations to do with the menstrual cycle may affect wake and sleep rhythms, making women more vulnerable to insomnia, sleep disturbances and tiredness. They may affect teenagers who are starting to menstruate and who may also have anaemia, which can itself affect sleep and therefore lead to more tiredness. Once menstruation is established, the pre-menstrual swings in levels of oestrogen and progesterone can cause pre-menstrual insomnia and sleep disturbance as part of pre-menstrual syndrome (PMS); while many are disturbed at night by the discomfort of menstruation itself, such as bloating, cramps and headaches. During pregnancy, women are often wakeful because of – depending on the trimester – nausea, backache, having to urinate, heartburn or their changed shape. Towards menopause, physical and hormonal changes take place that make sleep lighter, less deep and more likely to be broken. The heavier menstrual periods of later life may also bring anaemia.

Of course, for some women, hormonal issues are compounded or overshadowed by psychosocial factors. Many women cope with a paid job as well as with their roles as mothers and wives, and may cut back on their sleep, ignoring signs of fatigue as they put everyone else first. As we know, getting enough sleep has an enormous impact on a woman's life: it can make or break mood, and it can be the defining difference between just about managing, and being too tired to cope.

Pre-menstrual syndrome

Pre-menstrual insomnia and sleep disturbances during menstruation are just part of every month for some women. Although menstrual sleep disturbances have not received very much attention, the International Classification of Sleep Disorders includes pre-menstrual insomnia and the much rarer pre-menstrual hypersomnia (excessive sleepiness) as sleep disorders.

> Mair was losing four days each month because of insomnia and sleep disturbance, and she frequently had to take a day or two off work to cope. Unfortunately, the vicious cycle of exhaustion didn't end there – the poor sleep patterns tended to persist further into the month because she felt she had lost confidence in her ability to sleep. She partly solved the problem by deliberately staying up later and taking on more activities in the evenings, so that she was more physically tired when she went to bed, although the pre-menstrual time remained difficult in terms of sleep.

What happens is that the quality of sleep tends to worsen in the second half of the menstrual cycle as a result of rising progesterone levels. Sleep can also be disrupted before menstruation by symptoms such as tenderness in the breasts, bloating, headaches or mood swings, or by discomfort during menstruation itself, such as stomach cramps, raised temperature or excess blood flow. Cravings for food and alcohol before a period can also affect blood sugar levels, contributing both to fatigue and to any sleep difficulties. Coffee, alcohol and stress, as well as contributing to PMS, can also affect sleep, making it difficult to fall asleep and to stay asleep.

Even in women who do get enough sleep, extreme tiredness for a day or two is an unwelcome part of PMS for many women, hitting them every month, often suddenly, and sometimes being severe enough to make them take to their beds.

Although research in this area is rather lacking, there's some evidence to suggest that women who suffer from PMS have less deep sleep during the entire month, not just during the pre-menstrual week. The evidence suggests that it's best to try to treat pre-menstrual sleep difficulties holistically – that is, to tackle PMS itself all month long rather than isolating the sleep problem. Other symptoms of PMS include anxiety, headaches, weight gain, insomnia, bloating, irritability, breast tenderness, acne, moodiness, cramps and cravings for carbohydrates and sweets – certainly enough to justify taking the holistic approach!

No one is quite sure what causes PMS. One theory is that some women may be more sensitive to the hormone proges-terone released into the blood during the second half of the menstrual cycle, and one effect of progesterone is reduced levels of serotonin, the brain chemical involved in controlling mood and appetite. Low levels of serotonin can result in mood changes, irritability, sleep and cravings for carbohydrates. Some researchers also suspect that PMS is associated with fluctuating levels of calcium and vitamin D during the cycle.

Advice on diet in pre-menstrual syndrome

Again, thinking about what you eat and drink can make a huge difference to PMS. A balanced diet using foods with a low glycaemic index helps keep to blood sugar levels stable. Try to avoid caffeine, alcohol, sweets, biscuits and cakes; and be sure to eat every three hours to avoid blood sugar drops, which can make you feel awful during PMS (see Chapter 9). Here are some specific tips.

- Take a daily magnesium and calcium supplement (that is, take it all month). Some women find extra milk or other dairy products helpful in the days before a period. Extra calcium can also be found in leafy green vegetables.
- Other recommended supplements – although studies show mixed results – include vitamin B6, vitamin E, gamma-linolenic acid, evening primrose oil and starflower oil.
- Listen to your body. Rest; take time out, away from people and away from your usual routine. Stresses and strains that we take on the chin the rest of the month can seem unbearable now, and part of the tension can be sheer desperation for time off, a break from responsibilities. Let them wait until your hormones resettle and your energy returns.
- Make sure you drink plenty of water and get regular exercise, all month long but especially during PMS. Exercise helps to promote better sleep, and gets the system going, so helping rid it of toxins. Exercise does not have to be rigorous – a walk in the fresh air can work wonders.
- Try to get some sunlight first thing in the morning, especially during PMS itself. If there is no sun, natural daylight is better than nothing.
- Do ask your GP for advice if these simple measures don't work.

Pregnancy

Speculation abounds as to whether disturbed sleep during pregnancy is nature's way of starting to prepare an expectant mother for the reality of a new baby. However that may be, disturbed sleep during pregnancy is common – a 1998 survey by the National Sleep Foundation in the USA found that 80 per cent of pregnant women reported disturbed sleep, for a variety of reasons and depending on which trimester of pregnancy is in question. Pelvic pressure, lower back pain, the baby moving and pressure on the bladder were all reported as common factors.

During pregnancy, your body undergoes dramatic changes. For example, the amount of blood pumped by the heart increases by around 40 per cent and the size of the heart itself appears to increase by about 12 per cent, while your blood volume doubles. You are, after all, making a new person.

In the first trimester, higher progesterone levels may contribute to extreme fatigue and disturbed sleep. In addition, morning sickness can cause women to wake earlier than normal. During the second trimester, heartburn can become problematic, as can restless legs syndrome (see p. 67). In the third trimester, a woman's changed shape can make it difficult to find a comfortable position, and she may also be awoken by the baby kicking. The size and weight of the baby also slow her down, and fatigue tends to return.

Many women also find that they dream more vividly in pregnancy, owing to increased progesterone levels and the process of adjusting to the reality of the new situation. Common themes of these dreams include journeys; losing, searching and finding; doll babies; and babies that are smaller than normal or changed in shape. Again, this can be understood as the mind adjusting itself to the profound impending change in life.

Tiredness itself is also part of pregnancy – indeed, irresistible, overpowering fatigue is often its first sign, and some women continue to be shattered for the first three months. Older mothers, and those who are having a second, third or consecutive baby, may be more aware of fatigue. Tiredness tends to lift in the second trimester, often to return in the third – again, perhaps a safety measure of nature's – although some women do unfortunately just remain exhausted throughout pregnancy.

Although it's temporary, too many missed nights and too much tiredness can get some women down, so, even though some tiredness is natural in pregnancy, there are steps you can take to boost your energy.

- Most women have their iron levels checked during pregnancy but it may be worth having yours done again if you are feeling very drained. Check that your diet provides iron, which is found in red meat, fortified breakfast cereals, eggs, baked beans and other pulses, green leafy vegetables such as spinach and broccoli, dried apricots and prunes, and wholegrain breads and cereals.
- Eat the best possible diet you can. Discuss supplements with your doctor.
- Keep hydrated, and keep cool in hot weather.
- Nap when you can. Take as much rest as you can. Let chores go, or get others to help with them; get people to visit you, rather than you going out to see them.
- Keep up what exercise you can; many women find swimming enjoyable, especially as pregnancy progresses, because their buoyancy in the water brings relief from their extra weight. Yoga classes for pregnant women may also help.
- Talk to your doctor if insomnia persists or if you feel exhausted.

Childbirth

Giving birth is likely to be one of the most exhausting (and rewarding) experiences of your life. Do plan in as much rest as possible afterwards – don't try and 'get back to normal'. Again, eat the best possible diet you can, and nap when your baby does – don't, don't rush off to do the washing up.

Post-natal depression

Significant sustained tiredness along with weepy spells, irritability and feelings of depression or despair may signal post-natal depression. This isn't the 'baby blues', which is more or less a good howl some three or four days after the birth, but longer-lasting lowness of mood. One important symptom is feeling that you just can't cope. Do see your doctor as soon as possible because it is treatable.

Breastfeeding

Breastfeeding, although it is best for your baby, as well as helping you to lose that pregnancy weight, is physically draining. Again, it helps to eat a really good diet, including plenty or iron-rich foods, and to keep topped up with fluid yourself. Once you've given your baby a good start in life, though, if you do find breastfeeding very tiring, then it is not the end of the world if you want to supplement breastfeeding with a bottle, or to change to the bottle altogether.

Menopause

Menopause is defined as being one year from the last menstrual period.

The run-up to menopause – the perimenopause – can last some years and is a time when hormonal fluctuations increase, again causing fatigue. Sleep may also be disturbed by hot flushes and night sweats. Perimenopause is a time when periods often become heavier, so making anaemia – and tiredness – more likely. Again, a simple blood test can test your iron levels.

As with PMS, tiredness during menopause and before may be your body's natural way of asking for more rest. This is usually a full time of life for women, who may be at the height of their careers, with both teenage children and ageing parents needing attention, as well as a lifetime of accumulated plans, projects and expectations. When tiredness strikes at this stage, there is often a lot at stake; perhaps too much. Now may be a time when you need to reconsider priorities and goals in life, and what may need to be released: have a look at Chapter 5.

Much is made of hormonal shifts during menopause and their responsibility for fatigue. Many women get their energy back with hormone replacement therapy (HRT), but this doesn't work for everyone, and many women are concerned about side effects. Discuss the options with your doctor, and have a look at *Is HRT for You?* by Dr Anne MacGregor (Sheldon Press, 2003).

8

Sleep

Getting a good night's sleep, not just now and then but regularly, should be the foundation of your attack on fatigue. Population surveys in the UK and the USA indicate that as many as three-quarters of the adult population feel that they get insufficient or inadequate sleep. Doctors see only a small proportion of that number. The importance of sleep to health is receiving more attention, and there is a lot of media chat about what a sleep-deprived nation we are in our 24/7 society. Studies – particularly in the USA – worry away about how we get less sleep now than of yore and what a huge sleep debt we are accumulating, while other research has found links between poor sleep and obesity, depression, lowered immunity and heart disease. Sleep deprivation has also been linked with poor productivity and management, leading to irritability and mistakes – a survey by the think tank Demos found that 39 per cent of adults suffered from lack of sleep, rising to about 50 per cent among managers and those with young children.

On the other hand, a huge study by scientists at the University of California suggested that long sleepers die younger than do those who sleep fewer hours. The study of 1.1 million people found that those who sleep eight hours or more died younger (as do those who only managed four or less hours a night); however, six or seven hours a night was found to be condu-cive to a longer life. Another 25-year study at Southampton University involving 1,229 men and women also found that those who slept longer died younger.

So what is going on? Whom do we believe? Is less more in the battle against tiredness? Should we be sleeping six hours a night, or 10? And, given that we can't force ourselves to sleep, what's the point of arguing about it anyway? Surely it's an academic question? In fact, it's not clear exactly that longer sleep itself is related to earlier mortality, and some experts have suggested that the earlier mortality in these studies could be due to factors unrelated to sleep; one such expert is Professor Jim Horne of the Sleep Research Centre, Loughborough University, who is the author of *Sleepfaring: A Journey Through the Science of Sleep* (Oxford University Press, 2006). For example, many people who habitually sleep less than six hours are more likely to be heavy smokers, to have high-fat and low-fibre diets, to drink more alcohol, to do little exercise and generally to disregard their health. They might also be more stressed and desire more sleep.

Why we need sleep

Adequate sleep is as basic a biological need as food, water and air. Sleep deprivation has its most profound effects on the brain, and experiments in human beings show that a lack of sleep quickly leads to the slowing up of thought processes, impaired judgement, mood disturbance and irritability, behaviour changes and fatigue. The simplest way to regard sleep is therefore as a process of rest and repair, during which the brain (mainly) and body (to some extent) make good the 'wear and tear' of the previous day. This theory is attractive because it makes commonsense, but it lacks evidence to support it. For example, measurement of the brain's electrical activity (in a test called an electroencephalogram or EEG) shows that during sleep the brain is highly active, at times even more so than when awake. The many purposes of sleep are not confined to the brain alone. Significant changes occur during sleep in hormone levels, blood pressure and kidney function, for example. We do indeed seem to have an internal biological clock and we function best when this runs smoothly.

Lack of sleep

Sleep then remains something of a mystery in that we still don't really know exactly what it does do; it is, however, believed to serve several life-preserving functions. Laboratory animals deprived of sleep die within weeks – all complex animals need sleep, including the common fruit fly! In humans, we see how valuable sleep is by its lack: lack of sleep can cause headaches, tiredness and irritability, and generally cut down on your ability to function well.

Serious or ongoing lack of sleep can impair growth, because growth hormone is released during sleep, and it can seriously affect concentration and decision-making. It also weakens the immune system – one study found that lack of sleep is more damaging to the immune system than eating poorly, smoking or drinking. The research at the Department of Psychology at the University of British Columbia measured the body's production of antibodies, which fight infection. Studies at the Northwestern University, Chicago, also showed that insufficient sleep can impair the immune system.

Sleep deprivation can also cause or worsen stress, anxiety, depression and other mental health problems, cause hallucinations and antisocial behaviour, and reduce sex drive.

With continued lack of sufficient sleep, the part of the brain that controls language, memory, planning and the sense of time is severely affected, practically shutting down. In fact, 17 hours of sustained wakefulness leads to a decrease in performance equivalent to a blood alcohol level of 0.05 per cent (two glasses of wine) – the legal drink driving limit in the UK.

There are several suggestive studies that link lack of sleep with other key functions such as our cardiac health and the way we metabolize food.

Lack of sleep and heart disease

A study published in the *Archives of Internal Medicine* found that long-term sleep deprivation can boost a woman's risk of coronary heart disease, and that women who get five hours of sleep a night are 40 per cent more likely to have heart problems than those who sleep eight hours.

Lack of sleep and weight gain

Lack of sleep may also be a factor in obesity. In 2004, a study of more than 6,000 people conducted at Columbia University in New York found that people who sleep for two to four hours a night are 73 per cent more likely to be obese than those who sleep for seven to nine hours, and that those who sleep for five hours are 50 per cent more likely to be obese. It was found that people who slept a four-hour night had significantly decreased levels of the hormone leptin, which helps to regulate appetite and, in particular, signals to the brain that our bodies are full after eating. Researchers from the Case Western Reserve University in Ohio followed nearly 70,000 women for 16 years. They found that women who slept five or fewer hours a night were a third more likely to put on at least 15kg (33lb) than sound sleepers during the time of the study. It was suggested that sleep deprivation alters the balance of hormones that control the rate at which we burn off calories.

Lack of sleep and diabetes

Studies at the University of Chicago, Illinois, also link metabolic changes and sleep deprivation. They found that poor sleepers had lower levels of glucose tolerance, a measure of the body's ability to deal with blood sugar or glucose, which can lead to the early features of type 2 diabetes.

Don't worry too much!

Although severe and sustained sleep deprivation should indeed be attended to, the results of such studies do need to be treated with caution. Certain practical implications must also be weighed in the equation; as Jim Horne points out, a longer waking day also means more time in which to eat! And people who are too tired to exercise are more likely to gain weight, and so compromise their heart health; exhausted people may also find it easier to reach for a ready meal or convenience foods that are high in fat or sugar, again paving the way for heart disease and diabetes. So, while it is obviously important to get enough sleep on a regular basis, please don't lie awake worrying. Look at the suggestions for a good night's sleep below and, if you're really concerned, do visit your doctor.

Sleep and safety

Sleep deprivation doesn't just affect us; it also has an impact on others, especially if it happens regularly. An obvious and well-documented example is driving when tired, which is a factor in 20–30 per cent of accidents. For example, French researchers from the Centre Hospitalier Universitaire, Bordeaux, concerned at their country's high road accident rate, analysed 67,671 car crashes and found that fatigue, especially when combined with alcohol, presents a particularly high risk of road crashes resulting in death or serious injury.

Sleep deprivation has also been linked with major disasters such as the Space Shuttle *Challenger* disaster in 1986, The Bhopal gas leak in 1984, and the Chernobyl explosion in 1986. Moreover, one-third of accidents in several industries had sleep deprivation as an underlying cause, found Melissa Hack, Honorary Senior Lecturer in Sleep Medicine for the University of Wales. Her research found that the 24-hour economy is disrupting people's sleep rhythms without proper information on the effects of sleep deprivation, placing workers at risk of accidents, injury and depression.

Quantity of sleep: are we sleeping less than our ancestors?

In fact, not everyone believes that we are as sleep-deprived as it appears. Sleep experts such as Jim Horne believe that people sleep as much as circumstances allow them to. A free Sunday morning, with nothing to do, is conducive to a lie-in, in a way that having to catch the 6.37a.m. is not. One study showed that if people stay in bed two hours longer than in their normal routine, they will on average sleep for an extra hour – but because they have the opportunity to do so, not because they are sleep-deprived. Jim Horne cites the Inuit who, until they began to live a Westernized life in the 1950s, slept for as much as 14 hours on winter nights, but have adapted to a mere seven or eight.

There is a common perception that 'in the old days' people lived calmer, less stressful lives, and slept longer, in tune with the rising and setting of the sun. However, according to Jim Horne, the golden age of sleep is a myth. In fact, people may well have slept less in Victorian times, especially the working classes, because of longer working hours and poorer living conditions; five children to a bed, for example, or lack of central heating is not conducive to restful sleep. This is just as well, as the Victorians regarded more than seven hours sleep as self-indulgent, an attitude that's come down to us as part of our self-congratulatory work ethic. A survey for the Royal Mail by Melvyn Hodgetts on driver fatigue showed that 94 per cent of us 'do not consider getting enough sleep as important'. As the Royal Mail survey comments dryly, 'those that sacrifice their sleep on the altar of achievement are often admired.'

How much sleep?

It's generally agreed that between seven and nine hours of sleep a night is enough for most people. School-age children and teenagers need at least eight to ten hours of sleep, and often go short, with detrimental results to their mood, behaviour and performance.

Women may need more sleep than men. At the Sleep Research Laboratory at Loughborough University, a study involving 400 men and women found that women slept an average of seven and a half hours, about 15 minutes longer than men. Other studies suggest women need up to an hour's extra sleep a night compared with men, and not getting it may be one reason why women are much more susceptible to depression than men.

Losing just two hours of usual sleep requirement nightly over two weeks has been shown to cause the symptoms of fatigue in healthy subjects and significantly increases the likelihood of accidental injury.

Up to 95 per cent of people who have chronic fatigue syndrome report that sleep does not make them feel refreshed, and they may need to speak to their doctor about this. Up to 80 per cent of people, or more, with significant depression have disturbed sleep, typically wakening during the early hours of the morning.

Bear in mind that if you're tired, you may need more sleep than average for a while, until you feel better. However, don't worry too much about the exact number of hours. Quality of sleep can be even more important than quantity. Given the choice between a solid six hours of sleep and a broken eight, the tired person would probably opt for the former, to avoid the hung-over feeling that results from a disordered night's sleep.

Many sleep experts say that the body naturally takes what sleep it needs, catching up through naps if necessary. Expert opinion is also divided on whether a 'sleep debt' exists and, if so, whether sleeping more is the best way to pay it off. Generally, sleeping in at weekends is rather frowned on in the world of sleep experts, some of whom tend to tut-tut about the fact that a lie-in doesn't make up for a week of sleep-deprived nights – what a shame!

Daytime sleepiness

Sleep experts agree that the key clue to as to whether you're getting enough sleep is daytime alertness. If you are alert throughout the day, then you are probably getting enough sleep. Clues that you may not be not getting enough sleep include energy dips around lunchtime and around 4p.m.

This is all fine, unless you happen to be tired most of the time. The feeling of being alert throughout the day is precisely what tired people miss and long to regain. Furthermore, tired people who have a poor night's sleep, or who habitually sleep badly, don't just 'lack alertness' – they feel like walking zombies; they feel ill, 'out of it' or hung-over. If you habitually feel like this – punch-drunk after a bad night, rather than, or in addition to, feeling tired and lacking in energy – bear in mind that this can also be the profile of someone with a sleep disorder (see below). Sleep disorders are not just confined to the night, but are a 24-hour phenomenon. If this is you, do check out this kind of persistent 'walking-zombie' fatigue with your doctor.

Common sleep disruptors

Three main culprits in sleep disruption are:

- mental factors – stress, anxiety and depression;
- caffeine – it stays in the system for several hours, so even caffeine taken early in the day can adversely affect sleep;
- alcohol – it may help you drop off, but two standard servings of alcohol can reduce sleep by an hour; because it's a stimulant, it's more likely to wake you up again in the lighter stages of sleep.

Caring is a growing fourth factor – caring either for older relatives or for young children. In their survey, the think tank Demos found that the most common reason for loss of sleep was children waking. Worry about work, noisy neighbours and noisy traffic were also blamed.

Some research has singled out work time as the single most important lifestyle factor that has an impact on sleep – the more hours you work, the less sleep you get, according to the study in the journal *Sleep*, which included nearly 50,000 US participants and was conducted by Dr Mathias Basner of the University of Pennsylvania and colleagues. Those who got less than four and a half hours sleep a night worked an average of 93 minutes longer on weekdays and 118 minutes longer at the weekend. Commuting time ranked second – above socializing and leisure time – for eating into sleep time. Not only does work itself (and commuting) eat into relaxation time, it also leaves the person keyed up and so less likely to be able to unwind and sleep during the time he or she does have free.

Snoring, sleep apnoea and other sleep disorders

In recent years there has been increasing recognition of how sleep disorders such as sleep apnoea or restless leg syndrome can seriously disrupt sleep and cause chronic fatigue during the day. A good clue is that you can't remember the last time you woke up refreshed after a good night's sleep. If so, do consult your doctor.

Sleep apnoea is when breathing stops briefly during sleep; loud snoring and gasping are classic symptoms. Although sleep apnoea is traditionally viewed as a man's problem, it's now increasingly being recognized that it affects women too. Men are more susceptible as they tend to accumulate more fat around the neck as they age – which can obstruct breathing – and have narrower air pipes than women. However, many women gain fat in the neck after menopause, while younger women who are overweight also accumulate fat around the neck. Losing weight or sleeping on your side may help, but otherwise get advice from your GP if you suspect you have sleep apnoea or if snoring is a problem, because there are treatments available through sleep specialists.

Another sleep disorder is restless legs syndrome, twice as common in women than men, which is characterized by a creepy or crawly sensation in the legs. Restless legs can be associated with low levels of iron, which may be caused by heavy menstruation or pregnancy, or by a very strict vegetarian diet. Your doctor can test for low levels of iron and, if you do experience this, do avoid extreme dieting that may put you at risk of iron deficiency.

The Epworth Sleepiness Scale

The Epworth Sleepiness Scale is used to measure daytime sleepiness. It can help diagnose sleeping problems such as sleep apnoea.

How likely are you to doze off or fall asleep in the following situations in contrast to just feeling tired? Use the following scale to choose the most appropriate number for each situation. Even if you have not done some of these things recently, try to work out how they would have affected you. Here is the scale:

0: would never doze or fall asleep in this situation;
1: slight chance of dozing or falling asleep in this situation;
2: moderate chance of dozing or falling asleep in this situation;
3: high chance of dozing or falling asleep in this situation.

Situations (score each 0–3):
- sitting and reading;
- watching TV;
- sitting inactive in a public place; for example, in the theatre or at a meeting;
- as a passenger in a car for an hour without a break;
- lying down to rest in the afternoon when circumstances permit;
- sitting and talking to someone;
- sitting quietly after a lunch (without having drunk any alcohol);
- in a car, while stopped for a few minutes in traffic.

As a guide, a total score of 9 or more may mean that you have a sleep disorder such as sleep apnoea. See your doctor if you have a high score – and certainly if you do ever nap at the wheel – to discuss the results and your symptoms.

Heartburn and reflux

Reflux disease (also known as gastro-oesophageal reflux disease, or GORD) can cause persistent heartburn and lead to considerable discomfort at night. If you are overweight, then the main treatment is to lose weight; smokers should also stop smoking. Some people find it helps to eliminate spicy or acidic foods, which cause heartburn or indigestion at night.

Women and sleep

Women sleep more lightly and wake more easily than men, research indicates. They are in fact twice as likely as men to have difficulties falling asleep or staying asleep. However, sleep experts say that although it may be normal for women have more interrupted sleep than men, they are not immune to the dangers of disrupted sleep.

Young children, fluctuating hormones and stress are leading sleep thieves, according to Dr Kathryn Lee, a professor in the School of Nursing University of California, San Francisco, who found that 60 per cent of women get fewer than one or two nights of good sleep each week and that 40 per cent have sleep problems every night.

Hormonal fluctuations, it appears, affect women at virtually any stage of reproductive life (see Chapter 7). However, psychosocial problems may be more important than hormones. For some women, the question is: how much are they allowed to sleep – by the culture, their families, themselves?

Sleep reflects life

Sleep, like tiredness itself, reflects your life, health and lifestyle. Your sleeping style can reflect volumes about you, from whether you fall into bed like a contented log and slumber soundly all night, or whether you put off bedtime far beyond your natural rhythm because you're too busy and stressed rushing round preparing packed lunches, listening out for a baby, ironing clothes for tomorrow and shooing children into their beds. Babies are, of course, a special case; research shows that women wake more quickly than men when a baby cries, although experts disagree whether this is biological priming, and some suggest that, were a man alone with a baby, he'd wake up just as quickly.

More generally, today's lifestyle seems to leave women too wound up and overtired to sleep – even if they have time.

Sleep and exercise are the first things to go when women have too much to do in a day, according to a study at the University of California, San Francisco – a clear demonstration of how research confirms what we always knew. (The last to go is work.) Several studies have shown that many women cut down on sleep, ignoring tiredness in order to cope with work and their roles as mothers, wives and, increasingly, carers of elderly parents.

The National Sleep Foundation study revealed just how bad women are at giving in to tiredness – the vast majority, nearly 80 per cent, reached for a shot of caffeine if they felt tired, and just kept going. So, while tips about sleep hygiene are important, first consider your overall life situation, especially if you are a working mother.

Waking in the night or early in the morning

Waking early every morning – at, say, 4a.m. – and not being able to go back to sleep is classic insomnia, and may persist because the body clock becomes sensitized after waking up once or twice at that hour. Depression, stress or fluctuating hormones may be to blame.

One key reason for waking up at night is hunger – or, more precisely, a drop in blood sugar, which in turn stimulates the production of adrenaline, a stress hormone that will keep you awake and alert. In this case, a light snack such as a piece of fruit or a plain biscuit will help restore blood sugar levels. To prevent it happening, eat four to six small, well-balanced meals throughout the day to keep your blood sugar and energy levels steady (and also to prevent cravings). Have a light supper, not too soon before bedtime, to avoid being disturbed by digestive problems or the need to urinate – the traditional milky drink and carbohydrate snack is fine. Try a wholemeal sandwich, or a couple of plain biscuits; a baked potato helps keep blood sugar and serotonin levels steady throughout the night.

If the worst happens and you find you can't get back to sleep, don't worry; sit up, put the light on, get comfortable and read, listen to music, or write down any worries so they're off your mind. Get up and have a light snack or a warm bath, or tackle tasks such as ironing. Go back to bed when you feel tired again.

Night doesn't just happen

Preparing for sleep – what sleep experts call sleep hygiene – can make a huge difference to the quantity and quality of sleep. We are creatures of habit – go to bed at 10.05p.m. twice running, and you're fixed for life. More seriously, research shows that if you vary sleep and wake times more than 90 minutes, your sleep–wake cycle can be disrupted.

The good news is that sleep experts say that a huge amount of insomnia can be cured by easy – not to say obvious – self-help means, such as going to bed at the same time every night to regularize your biological clock, making sure your room isn't too hot or cold, and that (in case you hadn't thought of this one too) your mattress is comfortable. So, sleep well!

Sleep well

Daylight

Try to get some daylight, outside, first thing in the morning to regulate the body's production of melatonin, the hormone that helps to govern our sleep patterns. By providing a light signal in the morning and thus shutting down any melatonin release, you will enhance your ability to turn the melatonin back on at night. This helps you fall asleep faster and, ideally, stay asleep longer.

Wind down

This is especially important for busy working women, who may find their evenings swallowed by household and family cares. Try to make time for yourself – be selfish and shut the bedroom door if necessary. Read, write letters or note any anxieties or plans in a journal, to be put into action the next day. Don't do anything that will get the mental juices going or stir anxiety, like paying bills or trying to do your child's homework. Don't watch TV in your bedroom, don't have a computer in it, and make the bedroom yours, not somewhere for the rest of the family to invade. Banish the abandoned toys and the sports gear strewn everywhere, have a few favourite objects around such as ornaments, cushions, cosy socks – anything that proclaims this is your room to rest in.

Dietary and other considerations

Try a magnesium and calcium supplement. Magnesium has a soothing effect on the nervous system and is one nutrient that tends to be deficient in our diets; magnesium-rich foods include green leafy vegetables, beans, pulses and nuts. Calcium, found in dairy products, dark leafy green vegetables, baked beans and fortified cereals, also helps strained nerves to relax at bedtime. This supplement may be especially helpful just before and during menstruation, helping to soothe insomnia and other menstrual sleep difficulties, but take it all the month round.

Avoid alcohol and caffeine.

Consider any allergies – allergies to dust mites can make for uncomfortable nights, so consider a hypoallergenic mattress.

A bedtime snack helps to avoid blood sugar levels dropping in the middle of the night. Carbohydrates such as bread or cereal simulate the production of the hormone serotonin, which helps to induce sleep. Or try Dr Kathleen DesMaisons's tip and eat a baked potato two to three hours before bedtime to improve serotonin levels and help to prevent blood sugar dips and cravings for carbohydrates.

Certain foods contain a substance called tryptophan, which also helps to make serotonin. Foods high in tryptophan include eggs, lean meat, nuts, beans, fish, turkey, oats, bananas and milk – this is maybe one reason why bread and milk used to be such a popular Victorian supper for children. Milk contains calcium and tryptophan; bread, being a carbohydrate, would encourage the production of serotonin. Sleep handed to you on a plate (or in a bowl).

Avoid spicy foods and heavy meals, which can interfere with digestion and so disrupt sleep.

Another sleep-promoting snack is lettuce! Its traditional soporific properties, as noted by Beatrix Potter, do have a biological basis. Lettuce contains a substance called lactur carium that helps promote sleep by sedating the nervous system.

How to nap

A short nap – up to 20 minutes – has been shown to improve alertness (a longer one tends to leave you groggy). Research shows a 15-minute nap is more effective than a cappuccino at beating tiredness during the day, and sleep experts merrily advise a short nap in the middle of the day. That's great, but how do you manage one if you're surrounded by demanding toddlers or in the middle of an open-plan office, or if you just don't have the cat-napping temperament? It may help to view it more as meditation and a profound tuning-out from the world. Listening to music or white noise with headphones may be helpful. Just give yourself 10 minutes off, breathing slowly and deeply.

Your doctor

Some people's fatigue is not alleviated even by the best sleep routine, but this doesn't imply that the tiredness is then not worth investigating; on the contrary. So, if you are persistently having trouble sleeping even after trying the tips above, or if you still feel tired even if you do get enough sleep, do visit your doctor, who can make sure that your sleeplessness is not being caused by a sleep disorder, an undetected physical illness, a prescribed medicine or depression.

Medications for sleep problems

Sleeping pills are risky for many reasons. They don't treat the root cause of a sleep problem, and they can ultimately exacerbate insomnia. They interfere with deep sleep, and their sedative effects can extend into the daytime. Some are addictive or cause dependence for some people, and you may also develop a tolerance to them and need larger and larger doses. If you are having problems with sleeping pills, have a look at another Sheldon book, *Tranquillizers and Antidepressants: When to Take Them, How to Stop*, by Professor Malcolm Lader (2008).

Other commonly prescribed medications can also interfere with sleep. Don't forget also to check your over-the-counter medications – if in doubt, ask your doctor or pharmacist.

Instead of sleeping pills, try traditional methods to help you relax, such as lavender oil in your bath or on your pillow. The herb valerian has been found in studies to reduce the amount of time it takes to get to sleep, and it improves sleep quality. It is not addictive and appears to be relatively free of side effects.

In some cases, though, with your doctor's help, the careful use of the right medication can help to break sleep difficulties and need not cause trouble in the longer term. Certainly, however, the first approach should be without drugs, using the sorts of tips outlined already. Often people neglect these self-help measures, because they don't feel confident that such simple tricks can work. It's true that a half-hearted approach to them will usually fail, but taken together they can be quite successful.

When medication is necessary a wide range of drugs can be used.

Benzodiazepines

Examples of benzodiazepines are temazepam, nitrazepam and diazepam. These medicines help you to get off to sleep and have been in use for decades. They are effective and they have few direct side effects, but they do have addiction potential. One gets used to them very quickly (in two to three weeks), at which point their effect starts to wear off. This can lead to escalating dosage, which is undesirable. Coming off benzodiazepines may be difficult if they have been used continuously for more than a few weeks because of withdrawal effects, one of which is insomnia. Despite the disadvantages these drugs are still widely prescribed and are useful medicines when used for short spells.

Newer hypnotics

Zopiclone, zolpidem and zalepon are newer hypnotics, all of them short-lasting. These drugs possibly cause less trouble with dependence than the benzodiazepines but they are not free of the risk.

All of these hypnotic drugs are licensed for short-term use only because of the dependence potential. However, sleep disturbance does not tend to be a short-term problem, and many people stay on hypnotics for much longer than the recommended lengths of time. This is a very difficult problem, to resolve, because one is trying to help one problem while avoiding the creation of another. Not everyone has problems coming off hypnotics but it is best to avoid getting into difficulty if possible. This means limiting the use of hypnotics to short spells of two to three weeks maximum and then taking a break for a while. This can maintain the effectiveness of the drug and avoid dependence.

Antidepressants

Prior to the arrival of fluoxetine and drugs like it (collectively called the selective serotonin reuptake inhibitors, or SSRIs), the main drugs used for depression were the 'tricyclic' type of antidepressant. These tricyclic drugs are by no means obsolete although they are not now first choice for depression. One of the side effects of the tricyclic drugs was their tendency to sedate; however, this was partly an advantage if people with depression also had trouble sleeping – which commonly is the case. Examples of tricyclic antidepressants that are still in common use and that are sedating are amitriptyline, dosulepin and trimipramine.

Tricyclic antidepressants can therefore be used as aids to sleep but they also have disadvantages. They do not increase the amount of deep sleep that a person has and so, while they can help people to get off to sleep, they tend not to prevent people still waking in the morning feeling tired. Also, their side effects, such as a dry mouth, constipation and daytime drowsiness, can limit their use. The dose needed to aid sleep is, however, less than the dose needed for relief of depression, so with a bit of careful prescribing one can sometimes get a useful result without too many other problems. A big plus is that they are not addictive and do not cause dependence.

Most of the newer antidepressants, such as the SSRIs, are not sedative. They ultimately lead to an improvement in sleep in someone who is depressed by lifting the underlying depression, but this will not necessarily apply in people with persistent fatigue.

Mirtazapine and trazodone are more recent sedative antidepressants, and they can promote better quality sleep than the tricyclics – trazodone perhaps more so. They also have the advantage of not causing dependence. A low dose of trazodone is therefore an alternative to a benzodiazepine.

9

Nutrition

The key to nutrition is to keep it simple. Eat fresh, whole foods regularly. Avoid white sugar and flour. Cut down on alcohol and caffeine. Ignore faddy advice about 'super-foods' and very restricted diets, and make sure you have enough of certain key nutrients in your diet, including essential fatty oils, B vitamins, vitamin C, magnesium and calcium. Drink lots of water. And enjoy what you eat.

A tired body is crying out not just for food, but for nourishment. Too often, the exhausted person just eats what's there, or what's easiest, or what will feel most comforting – such as bread or biscuits. But if you wait a moment before reaching for comfort food, often you might find that in fact, in those few moments before eating, you are thinking of something quite different – grapes, say, instead of chocolate digestives, or kidneys instead of a bun.

This is especially true if you're exhausted by constant stress. Ongoing high levels of the stress hormone cortisol can cause you to crave carbohydrates and sugar, because one of cortisol's functions is to ensure the body gets enough fuel to withstand the next crisis. But, although the carbohydrate and sugar duo may give a surge of energy that's just right for an American pioneer building his family an emergency shelter against wolves before sunset, it isn't usually used up in any such violent exercise by us today. Instead, after the initial rise, blood sugar drops and you feel tired yet again.

So, next time you feel hungry, why not ask yourself what you are hungry for? Is it really sweets or crisps, or is your body asking for a fresh salad? A proper cooked hot meal? Are you even hungry for food? Maybe you need water, rest or recreation more? Sometimes the body interprets wishes as physical hunger, but quite a wide range of motives can disguise themselves as hunger.

Dehydration

Dehydration in particular is a surprisingly common cause of fatigue – in fact, tiredness rather than thirst is often the first sign of dehydration. For some reason, thirst itself is not a reliable sign of dehydration – you can't judge how dehydrated you are by how thirsty you feel. Often, by the time you feel thirsty, you are already somewhat dehydrated. Another early symptom of dehydration can be hunger, leading people to eat rather than drink. In short, many people don't realize just how dehydrated they are.

Even low levels of dehydration can make you tired. Losing just 2 per cent of body fluid is enough to cause a drop in energy levels, headaches, lack of concentration and short-term memory loss.

The main problem with dehydration is that the lack of water reduces blood volume, so that less blood – and so less oxygen – is available to the body. This has an adverse impact on organs such as heart, brain and kidneys, as well as on the digestive system: the less blood they have, and the less oxygen, the less able they are to function.

You should therefore aim to drink before you actually feel you need to, keeping your fluid levels topped up by sipping around eight glasses of water, herbal tea or diluted, unsweetened juice a day (not coffee or tea, because they are diuretic). Get into the habit of having fresh drinks of water around while you work, and don't forget to take a bottle of water with you when you go out.

Have breakfast

Tiredness and poor nutrition have a complex interlinked bio-chemical relationship. This starts in the morning with breakfast, which begins the job of keeping your blood sugar steady for the day. Blood sugar levels tend to drop overnight while you're asleep, and they are often low when you wake up. Breakfast helps to stabilize blood sugar levels, which in turn helps to regulate your appetite an and energy. In other words, if you start the day with breakfast, you are much more likely to feel hungry at the right times, and to be more energetic. Thinner, too, because breakfast also helps weight loss. Studies have consistently shown that those who miss breakfast eat more, not fewer, calories throughout the day, whereas breakfast is consistently associated with better weight control.

Sleeping itself burns 300–400 calories or more; this, added to the fact that in the morning your last meal is now several hours behind you, means that your system needs food in order to get going. Breakfast restarts the metabolism and sets the stage for a day of energy. When you skip breakfast, your metabolic rate slows down and your blood sugar drops. As a result, you become hungry and have less energy, setting the scene for impulsive snacking on junk food, or for eating more at lunch or dinner – which again leads to blood sugar dips and more tiredness.

Not having enough time is a common problem for many, especially tired people who long for another few minutes in bed, or who maybe haven't slept well at night and then need to sleep in a bit in the morning. Try setting the alarm 15–20 minutes earlier and having breakfast in bed. Or have a cup of tea and a couple of oatmeal or plain biscuits, and then do as the Germans do and have a *zweites Frühstück*, a second breakfast, later when you've reached work, taken the kids to school or just warmed up to the day a bit more. However, you might not want to follow the breakfast menu laid out in novelist Sybille Bedford's version of a second breakfast in Berlin, as described in her novel *A Legacy*, which includes venison with redcurrant jelly, potted meats, tongue, poussin, sweetbreads, smoked breast of goose and port wine.

A slightly later breakfast can also be helpful if you find you're not hungry first thing in the morning. Lack of appetite can also be helped by having breakfast at the same time every day – give it a few days to have an effect. Also try not to eat too late at night. Try to make your last meal or snack around two hours before bedtime.

Good choices for breakfast include wholegrain cereals, peanut butter on toast, cottage cheese and fruit, egg and a muffin – but basically, anything you fancy will help get the metabolism going. Try and stay away from sugary doughnuts, though.

Eat regularly

Eating three smallish well-balanced meals a day, with two or three healthy snacks, will go a long way to keeping levels of blood sugar and energy steady. It's important to exclude or limit foods that contain sugar and white flour. Keep portions modest – a huge meal can also leave you tired as energy goes into digestion.

Planned eating in this way prevents those awful mid-morning and mid-afternoon dips in energy when the temptation to grab a doughnut is at its highest; it also prevents the sag and fatigue in the early evening.

Marta's day finished at 5p.m. with the end of work. She would get home, grab a meal and flop into a chair, too exhausted to do anything for the rest of the evening. She would have a good breakfast, but typically snacked on crisps and a doughnut at 11a.m., then had an apple at lunchtime and nothing else for the rest of the day until she went home for her early evening main meal. Lately, too, she'd been noticing that her energy was running out earlier and earlier in the day – first at 3p.m., then even at 2p.m. By adjusting her food intake to five or six smallish meals a day, she found she had much more staying power. And, although she ate far more, she also lost a couple of pounds in the first two weeks.

Enjoy your food

This is especially important in fatigue, especially if you suspect you're tired because you've been under constant stress. As mentioned in Chapter 6 on stress, the stress response can 'shut down' the digestive system, making meals hard work and the digestive aftermath downright unpleasant.

Eating while stressed or angry is counterproductive. When the stress response is unleashed, what happens is that the body diverts blood supply and energy from other areas of the body, such as the digestive system.

A good, nutritious diet goes a long way towards soothing stress and rebalancing the hormones that may have got out of kilter in adrenal exhaustion. So, how and where you eat is important. It isn't a matter of grabbing a sandwich while you do something else. Meals, even small ones, should be enjoyable breaks where you can relax and know that by nourishing yourself you are giving yourself the best possible chance against fatigue and ill-health.

> Karen found she suffered acute stomach ache and wind all afternoon and evening if she ate at her desk at work or on the run at home. It was all part of a lifestyle where she was, she felt that she was 'running to stand still' and that she was constantly losing ground, and losing energy. When she learned deliberately to slow down, she began to feel much better. Part of this was taking half an hour out from whatever she was doing for a relaxed lunch with a book or magazine.

Which foods?

There are no magic foods. In magazine or web articles you may see lists of the latest 'super-foods' but, while they may be excellent foods in their own way, each food is only ever part of a healthy diet.

In general, if you think fresh and whole, you can't go far wrong, and probably what you exclude is as important as what you include. Certainly, most people can tell when they've eaten too much of the wrong kind of foods – they feel bloated, sluggish and fatigued.

False friends

Some foods are false friends – they promise energy but actually drag the body down. Three main culprits are discussed below.

Caffeine

Caffeine increases alertness and mental performance, and it is also widely proven to be what researchers call an ergogenic aid (that is, a substance that improves the capacity to do work or exercise). While small hits of caffeine may be a pleasant stimulus, excessive amounts can disrupt blood sugar levels, deplete the body of nutrients, prevent good sleep and cause fatigue. The key is moderation. Stick to two or three cups a day, and drink instant in preference to brewed coffee.

Some people are exceptionally sensitive to the effects of caffeine, finding they suffer sleep problems and other problems such as breast tenderness even after just one cup of coffee a day. Caffeine also remains in the system for several hours, so that even a strong coffee drunk in the morning may be enough to cause insomnia in some people. People sensitive to caffeine may find their fatigue definitely improves when they give it up completely. Bear in mind that ordinary tea contains caffeine, as do some fizzy drinks and energy drinks.

Sugar

Simple sugars, found in cakes, chocolate, sweets, pastries, biscuits, ice cream and refined processed food like white bread may give you a quick boost of energy, but they lead also to a quick drop in blood sugar levels.

Alcohol

Like sugar, alcohol causes swings in your blood sugar levels. It's best to exclude it, or to limit to no more than one drink a day.

Unhealthy fats

Saturated fat, found mostly in meat and full-fat dairy products, is another energy drainer you need to avoid. It's the major culprit in raising blood cholesterol, the main ingredient of artery-clogging plaque. Overindulging in these foods raises the risk of developing heart disease, weight gain and poor health, all of which will slow you down and wear out. You can lower this risk by shifting the emphasis so that nutrient- and fibre-rich foods such as fruits, vegetables and grains make up approximately two-thirds of what you eat each day. However, the right fats are very important – indeed some research suggests they have a key role to play in fatigue (see the discussion about essential fatty acids, below). A diet that is too low in fat, as well as depleting energy levels, also makes it harder to lose weight.

A word about salt

Salt – more specifically, sodium – is vital to adrenal health; indeed, one symptom of adrenal exhaustion can be salt craving due to sodium deficiency, symptoms of which include muscle weakness, poor memory and concentration, and dehydration. Given the amount of salt in most modern diets and in processed foods, most people consume not too little but too much sodium, and it's true that this leads to an increased risk of heart disease, stroke and high blood pressure, and kidney stones.

On the other hand, the body needs more than 100 milligrams of salt a day to function properly. So, if you usually eat a diet of whole, fresh foods, and know that you don't normally consume much salt, it's sometimes recommended that you try adding a little sea salt to your diet. However, don't overdo it and if in doubt see your doctor, who should really be the one to make a diagnosis of adrenal exhaustion in any case.

Food sensitivity and fatigue

Food sensitivity is a common accompanying complaint to those with chronic fatigue, and several studies have documented improvements in energy when the offending foods are given up. The most common food culprits are wheat, dairy products and sugar. The body uses a great deal of energy to digest these. So if your lunch was a cheese sandwich with a bar of chocolate, your body may be using up energy by simply digesting it rather than converting your lunch into energy.

Keep a food diary for a few weeks and see if there is a connection between your tiredness and a specific food. Try eliminating that food and see if it makes a difference. Alternatively, you can have a blood test to check for food allergies. A blood test will generally find only true allergies, however, not sensitivities. While it is common to confuse allergies and sensitivities, the latter are far more common. An allergic reaction to a food – such as an itchy or swollen mouth or throat, a rash or itchy or swollen skin, or a wheeze, cough or runny nose – usually occurs quite soon after eating the food, within the hour. A sensitivity or intolerance – with symptoms such as diarrhoea or constipation, wind, bloating stomach pain, migraine, or nausea and vomiting – is more likely to occur over hours or days.

Nutrients to include

Essential fatty acids

Omega-3 and omega-6 oils are essential fatty acids found in fish, nuts and seeds that are important for metabolism and healthy brain function; and tiredness is a major symptom of deficiency. There's also some evidence that extra essential fatty acids may help with persistent, established fatigue.

The UK Department of Health suggests that we should double our intake of omega-3 fatty acid by eating oily fish, such as salmon, mackerel, herrings and sardines, two or three times a week. Some research suggests that the oils are better absorbed from fish than from supplements. Other sources include nuts – especially walnuts – and seeds, whole grains, olive oil and sunflower oils, and linseed oil or flaxseed oil. Virgin evening primrose oil is another source of omega-6 fatty acid, and it is thought to help fatigue in some cases, although more research is needed on this, and the research that exists has produced conflicting results, with one study reporting benefit after 3 months of taking 4 grams daily and another, using the same dose, showing no benefit.

Flaxseeds

Flaxseeds themselves are a good source of omega-3 oils and also help prevent constipation; numerous other health benefits have been claimed for them too, including protection against heart disease, diabetes and cancer to name but a few. They are, however, difficult to eat, tending to stick to the teeth and also to pass undigested through the body. One idea is to let them 'soak' in some live yoghurt and eat them once they have softened and swelled, chewing well. Or grind them in a blender with fresh juice or a yoghurt smoothie, and drink at once.

Magnesium

Magnesium has a general sedating effect on the nervous system, and is one nutrient that tends to be deficient in our diets. It's also essential for energy production, and deficiency has been linked to fatigue and muscle weakness. Magnesium-rich foods include leafy green vegetables, beans, nuts, seeds, whole grains, broccoli, bananas and potatoes. You might also want to consider a supplement.

Potassium

Low levels of the mineral potassium may cause muscle weakness and tiredness. Good sources of potassium include fruit such as bananas, vegetables, pulses, nuts and seeds, milk, fish and shell-fish, beef, chicken and turkey, and bread.

Iron

Iron is a trace element that aids in energy production and is essential for proper immune functioning. Good sources of iron include high-quality meats and offal, poultry and fish, as well as seaweeds, nuts, sunflower seeds, pumpkin seeds, whole grains and leafy greens, especially kale and spinach.

B vitamins and vitamin C

If you eat a good, varied diet with plenty of fresh and whole foods, you are likely to have good sources of these vitamin groups. Both are important for energy and to beat stress.

Lack of the B vitamins cause fatigue; these vitamins help your body deal with stress and are vital for energy production. The B vitamins are found in meat (especially liver), poultry, yeast extract (such as Marmite and brewer's yeast), brown rice, wheat germ, whole grains, fish, nuts and pulses, dried fruit (such as apricots, dates and figs), vegetables (such as spinach, broccoli, asparagus and potatoes), milk, eggs, cheese, yoghurt and soybeans and soybean products. Vitamin C, a powerful antioxidant, is found in broccoli, cabbage, leafy greens, squash, red and green peppers, cantaloupe, strawberries, oranges and grapefruit.

A deficiency of folic acid, vitamin B, vitamin C, magnesium, potassium and zinc can lead to tiredness. If your energy levels are low, take a multivitamin and mineral supplement containing around 100 per cent of the recommended daily amount (RDA) of as many micronutrients as possible as a nutritional safety net to guard against deficiencies. This will give you a good combination of vitamins and minerals that are essential for energy production.

Vitamin B12 injections have long been used as a 'treatment' for fatigue and as an 'energy booster', both in human and in veterinary medicine. Vitamin B12 is essential for the body to manufacture red blood cells and for the maintenance of the 'insulating' material that covers nerves. It is absorbed from foods of animal origin and most people have no difficulty obtaining enough vitamin B12 from their diet – in fact, detectable deficiency is uncommon, although vegetarians and the elderly are at risk, as are those unable to absorb vitamin B12 from the intestinal tract (which causes pernicious anaemia). Unfortunately, while vitamin B12 has been used to treat established fatigue, existing trials don't really differentiate the real effect and the placebo effect strongly enough.

If you are worried about your level of B vitamins, it's best to increase your intake of foods rich in these vitamins, as listed above, and, if you do want to take a supplement, to make it a supplement of vitamin B complex to ensure you get a good balance of B vitamins.

Probiotics

As poor digestion leads to nutritional deficiencies and fatigue, some people find it helpful to take probiotics, supplements of 'friendly' bacteria that help balance digestion. Probiotics can be found in live natural yoghurt containing *Lactobacillus acidophilus* and in fermented food sauces such as miso, sourdough bread and sauerkraut.

Good gut bacteria can also be boosted by eating fruit and vegetables, which contain prebiotics – the sugars that nourish 'friendly' bacteria.

Take your time

All the diet recommendations in this chapter can make a significant difference to your energy levels and, if you've been having
trouble sleeping, they may also help you sleep better and wake
refreshed. It is important, though, to take your time incorpo-
rating any changes. For instance, if you aren't used to eating a
high-fibre, whole food diet, suddenly introducing lots of fibre
can lead to wind and indigestion. Likewise, if you've been used
to drinking 10 cups of coffee a day, it's best to decrease the
number gradually, because cutting back too quickly can lead to
withdrawal symptoms such as headache. Start by making small
changes.

Tiredness and weight gain

Tiredness and weight gain often go hand in hand. This can be
part of the whole stress syndrome, including factors such as
adrenal fatigue (see p. 48) and insulin resistance (see p. 19). Also
bear in mind that it's worth checking tiredness and unexplained
weight gain with your doctor, as they can sometimes indicate a
thyroid problem.

It's well documented that sustained weight loss is best achieved
gradually, and that it's best to think in terms of a long-term
healthy eating plan, with several sustained small changes, not in
terms of 'a diet'. Many tired people, however, find that they try
faithfully to eat sensibly, with plenty of fresh fruit and vegetables,
as advised, not too many cake and chocolate binges – but that
nothing happens. They have perhaps the comfort of not gaining
any more weight, but they don't lose as much as a pound. What
can be done in this situation?

- Try to re-evaluate your stress levels, because stress is a hidden
  trigger for weight gain.
- Eat six small meals or snacks a day, rather than three large

ones, and try to ensure that you eat more food in the first half of the day than in the second.

- Watch the salt content of your diet, because it can cause you to retain water.
- Cut out white flour in any form (bread, biscuits, pasta and so on).
- Be scrupulous about unnoticed calories from sauces, salad dressings and so on.
- Read the calorie content of anything you buy, including diet foods, low-fat yoghurts, and so on.

Weight gain in itself is a major cause of ongoing tiredness. To be blunt, our bodies weren't designed to bear the extra weight, which puts a strain on joints and organs such as the heart, and is tiring to carry around. Try taking a couple of bags full of heavy books into work with you, or when you next go for a walk, to appreciate how much the extra weight may put a strain on the system. At least you can put the weight of the books down at the end of the journey!

Overweight people also tend to suffer more from sleep apnoea and other sleep disorders, which also contribute to fatigue.

Too much weight also militates against the very activity that would help a person lose weight – exercising while overweight is tiring.

The suggestions in this chapter will help you get the proper balance with regard to food intake. Be especially sure to eat little and often to balance blood sugar and help prevent binge-eating. In addition, ensure you have enough sleep – sleep loss often militates against weight loss (see above).

There may also be an emotional factor in your eating pattern, in which case you may be able to get help from your doctor or a professional nutritionist or dietician. Have a look at *Coping with Compulsive Eating* by Ruth Searle (Sheldon Press, 2006).

Finally ...

Do eat enough. Be sure you are consuming enough calories. Some people, especially women, and especially women trying to lose weight, become tired simply because they don't eat enough. Being underweight also contributes to tiredness; indeed, if you're thin enough to be tired because of it, it could be quite a serious problem. If you have trouble gaining enough weight, again, you should consult your doctor or a nutritionist. At the extreme end of the spectrum is anorexia nervosa, a serious but treatable condition. If you suspect this, do take advice from your doctor, and ask to be referred to an eating disorders expert. Another Sheldon book that can help is *Overcoming Anorexia* by Professor J. Hubert Lacey, Christine Craggs-Hinton and Kate Robinson (2007).

The average woman should eat about 1,500 to 1,700 calories a day, and regular exercisers about 1,800 to 2,000. Consuming less than that may leave you feeling tired and irritable. If you do want to lose weight, take it slowly and aim for just one or two pounds a week and increase your exercise.

10

Activity and exercise

When you're really tired, even routine tasks like having a shower or washing up become an effort. And you tend to slow down. Tasks that should be easy become difficult, or take more time than they should, or take a long time to recover from – or any combination of the three. Sing the praises of 'exercise' all you want, but the tired person is unlikely to be fired up. Even the prospect of a 'nice brisk walk', so often put forward by doctors as a kind of last-ditch attempt to get people moving, may fail to appeal.

Enthusiasm for movement in general – as opposed simply to 'exercise', a word that always implies making an extra effort – tends to decrease in direct proportion to a person's tiredness. To use a favourite phrase of my grandmother's, the less you do, the less you want to do. Oversimplification though this is, there is some truth in it in cases of ordinary fatigue.

We know that just one week of resting in bed reduces your muscle strength by 10 per cent. The more unfit you become, the more tired you will be when you try to do something. The fitter you are, the better you can resist the invidious onslaught of tiredness. Everything – even driving a car – becomes easier, and less fatiguing, when you are fit. It's well documented that 'exercise' gives you more energy, building up energy and endurance. A fit person finds everything easier, from walking to school to picking up the kids, to running for the train or getting through a long day at work.

The benefits

Exercise gets your heart and lungs going, oxygenates your entire system and boosts your mood. Muscular movement gets toxins flowing through the body's lymph system to the liver and kidneys, whence they can be excreted by the body. By helping the body to eliminate stress hormones such as cortisol and adrenaline, exercise helps you relax and sleep better.

In a study published in the *Psychological Bulletin*, the researchers analysed 70 studies on exercise and fatigue involving more than 6,800 people. More than 90 per cent of the studies showed that sedentary people who completed a regular exercise programme reported improved fatigue compared with those who did not exercise. The average effect was greater than the improvement from using stimulant medications.

But, as stated, unfortunately tiredness itself militates against 'exercise'. The prospect of stepping out boldly in the competitive air of a gym alongside rather fit and rather energetic enthusiasts, or the whole paraphernalia of trying to go swimming in a public swimming pool on a cold morning, is almost guaranteed to turn off the average person suffering from tiredness. So why not keep it gentle to begin with, and have a long-term aim of building up your fitness and energy to the point where you can decide to take it further if you want to. The real aim is to build enough fitness to get through the average day and have a bit left over for emergencies – running for the bus or after a runaway toddler, driving out to pick up a stranded teenager at 11p.m. Or just feeling how nice it is to get to the end of the day and be pleasantly tired, rather than tumbling into bed at an early hour in a state of absolute exhaustion. Energy building, and energy conservation, ideally means having something in the bank, or keeping it in reserve, rather than having to spend it all as you go along.

Walking

Walking is an ideal way to get the system going, exercise muscles and get some fresh air at the same time. Try to build it up slowly on a day by day basis and don't worry if you don't get too far at first. Like losing weight, exercise is best done gradually, bit by bit. Walk halfway round the block today, and all the way round tomorrow. Don't push yourself. Almost any exercise, however small, is better than none, and if you build it up little by little, progress will be made, even if it is gradual.

Car dependence

Car dependence is a global health issue. Ian Roberts is professor of public health at the London School of Hygiene and Tropical Medicine. Writing in the *Guardian*, he points out how every day about 3,000 people die and 30,000 people are seriously injured in traffic accidents, many of them children and in developing countries. By 2020, road crashes are expected to move from ninth to third place in the world ranking of the burden of disease and injury, and they will be in second place in developing countries.

A report by Royal Automobile Club (RAC) underlines the increase in car dependency among UK residents. The study found that most motorists would be reluctant to switch to public transport, even if services were vastly improved. A massive 89 per cent of drivers surveyed said that they would find life 'very difficult' without a car. Yet, car travel has drastically reduced our walking, most shamefully on short journeys (less than two miles), which make up a quarter of all car journeys. Car dependence is a major factor in our growing obesity crisis and all its related health issues such as heart health, osteoporosis and diabetes. So if you do nothing else, try leaving the car home for short journeys; plan in more time for walking to your destination.

Try stretching your body

Eastern style exercises such as tai chi, chi chung and yoga are specially designed to build health and energy, to stretch muscles and to help you to eliminate toxins, and stretching exercises seem to work well for those with fatigue. If a class seems too much effort, a video can help you to exercise at your own pace in the comfort of your own home, where you can stop as soon as you feel tired. Yoga is particularly good for tiredness.

Yoga

Yoga is a centuries-old, effective way to boost energy. It also relaxes the body and mind, improves blood flow and oxygenation, stretches muscles, improves breathing and reduces tension. Writing in the journal *Neurology*, researchers in the Department of Neurology at Oregon Health and Science University reported that yoga significantly reduced fatigue in people with multiple sclerosis.

Many of the postures are designed to work on the hypothalamus, the master gland that controls the body's endocrine system, and to combat fatigue, notably the shoulder stand (see p. 28). If you are not a yoga devotee, however, begin with something gentler – breathing and gentle stretching exercises. (See also the exercises for yoga and the thyroid in Chapter 3.)

Relaxation breath

Sit up, with your back straight. Place your tongue behind your upper front teeth and keep it there throughout the exercise. Exhale completely through your mouth. Close your mouth and inhale through your nose to a count of four. Hold your breath for a count of seven. Exhale completely through your mouth, to a count of eight. Repeat this cycle three more times for a total of four breaths. Try to do this breathing exercise at least twice a day.

Deep diaphragm breath

Sit with your legs crossed in a comfortable position. Breathe slowly and evenly from your diaphragm, through your nose. Fill your lower abdomen, your lungs and then your chest with air. Hold for a four count then slowly exhale the air out from your chest, lungs and then the lower abdomen. Repeat three or four times.

Alternate nostril breathing

A great energizer, alternate nostril breathing synchronizes the left and right sides of the brain.

Close the right nostril with your right thumb and inhale through the left nostril to the count of four seconds. Then close the left nostril with your right index finger, simultaneously opening your right nostril and exhaling through it to a count of eight seconds. Now inhale through the right nostril to the count of four seconds. Close the right nostril with your right thumb and exhale through the left nostril to a count of eight seconds. Repeat three times.

Exercise tips

- Start low and work up slowly. Aim to build up exercise on a daily basis to comfortable levels, bit by bit. For example, if a 30-minute walk is too daunting, try a 10-minute one to start with, and build it up by five minutes a day.
- If that is too much, try, say, a five-minute walk a day, and stick with it for a week before increasing it.
- 'Exercise wipes me out.' Do listen to your body – if you're tired after exercise, take heed, and do less next time, until you do feel comfortable. But don't give up.
- Exercise slowly and rest afterwards.
- Keep track of how much exercise you do, and how it affects you, with an activity journal.

- Experiment – if you don't fancy stretching exercises or yoga, think about swimming or a gentle game of tennis, or a dance class. Housework also counts as activity and light exercise. Look for motivation – for example, a pet dog will make daily walking more of a reality!
- Stop before you feel tired – don't push yourself to the limit.
- If you don't feel up to exercising on a particular day, try to do some very gentle activity, but don't force yourself. Almost any exercise, however small, is better than none, but if nothing else, make sure you get some fresh air and daylight.

11

Complementary therapies

In practice, the things most likely to help with ordinary tiredness include:

- enough sleep;
- adequate nutrition – enough protein and fresh produce, less sugar, white flour, alcohol and caffeine;
- planned rest each day; and
- more exercise, built up at a comfortable level, especially in sunlight or daylight.

However, there are times when everyone needs a little more help, or it would be a drab life. So, if wanting an extra boost or kick start from a complementary therapy, where do you start?

In something as 'general' as tiredness, the field of complementary remedies is equally broad. Roughly, the theory behind many complementary remedies is that tiredness is caused by an imbalance in the body's natural energy flow, which the remedy helps to redress. Perhaps one of the joys of complementary remedies with regard to tiredness is that they sidestep the whole distinction between mind and body that has dogged efforts to treat fatigue. Ayurvedic medicine, for example, views fatigue as something that may result from both physical and mental stress – as well as from not enough stress, or boredom. Viewing fatigue from the mind–body–spirit perspective can help to focus on finding ways to manage and overcome the tiredness rather than feeling impelled to find a cause.

Reflexology

Reflexology is a form of foot massage designed to treat specific problems and to restore the flow of vital energy throughout the body. Reflexology is based on the concept of reflex points, located in the feet which correspond to all parts of the body, and practitioners believe that by manipulating these points the whole body can be treated.

Try the following to relieve stress and fatigue. Find a point about two inches below the middle toe, about a third of the way down the total length of the foot. Press deeply with your thumb for a minute or two, or massage just before going to bed.

Aromatherapy

Essential oils of jasmine, peppermint and rosemary are calming and restorative and may be used in aromatherapy. Place several drops in a warm bath or atomizer, or on a cotton ball. Other oils of interest include bergamot to revive, lemongrass to counter sluggishness, orange to lighten mood, rose to increase alertness, black pepper to overcome emotional blocks and mental exhaustion, and peppermint to give a physical and mental uplift.

Acupuncture

Anecdotal evidence points to good results for fatigue with acupuncture, an ancient Chinese method for treating pain. The treatment involves inserting very fine needles into acupuncture points in the body to redirect your Qi or vital energy into a more balanced flow. Breakthrough Breast Cancer are running a large clinical trial, The ACU.FATIGUE study, to investigate whether acupuncture may help women with breast cancer to cope with fatigue, a major side effect of breast cancer treatment.

Herbal remedies

If you are on medication, trying for a baby or have a pre-existing medical condition, consult your doctor before taking any herbs or supplements.

Siberian ginseng (*Eleutherococcus senticosus*), used in Asia for centuries to increase energy and fight tiredness, is often recommended to help the body cope during stress or after illness. A survey of 155 people with persistent fatigue conducted by researchers at the University of Iowa found that ginseng was considered one of the more helpful treatments, with 56 per cent of the people who used ginseng rating it as effective.

Another herb that may prove beneficial for tiredness is echinacea to support the immune system.

Liquorice has been used since ancient times as a food and a medicine and is a common ingredient in Chinese herbal medicine. It is often recommended for adrenal exhaustion, because the root is known to stimulate the adrenal glands and to block the breakdown of active cortisol in the body. While there have been no large clinical trials of liquorice in people with fatigue, some preliminary studies suggest it may be worth a try. Do not use liquorice if you have high blood pressure, oedema or heart problems.

Supplements

Carnitine

Carnitine (L-carnitine, or levocarnitine) is a nutrient found in the body that helps convert fatty acids into energy that used mostly for muscular activities. Low carnitine levels can result in fatigue. Lack of carnitine may be due to diet or to physical problems such as genetic disorders or liver or kidney problems. A small study of people with chronic fatigue syndrome showed improvement when they took extra carnitine. A Japanese study at the Osaka University Medical School also showed low carnitine levels in those with chronic fatigue syndrome.

Sources of carnitine include red meat (particularly lamb) and dairy products. Carnitine can also be found in fish, poultry, tempeh (fermented soybeans), wheat, asparagus, avocados and peanut butter. It's also available as a supplement.

Eicosapentaenoic acid

Research suggests that a supplement called eicosapentaenoic acid may be of benefit, especially when taken with virgin evening primrose oil. This is no more than our old friends the essential fatty acids – omega-3 oils (see Chapter 9).

Coenzyme Q10

Coenzyme Q10 (CoQ10) is an antioxidant naturally occurring in the body (and in small amounts in meat and seafood such as mackerel and herring), which provides cellular energy. While it is probably best known for its promoted role in heart health, a small study at the University of Iowa suggested that 69 per cent of people with chronic fatigue found CoQ10 helpful. Research also indicates that CoQ10 helps to boost athletic performance.

Coconut oil

There has been increasing interest in coconut oil as a possible treatment for a range of ills, including hypothyroidism, fatigue, diabetes, candidiasis, obesity, headache, digestive problems and more! The beneficial effect of coconut oil is thought to be due to its lauric acid, a medium-chain fatty acid that speeds up the metabolic rate and so helps weight loss and general energy. It also contains medium-chain triglycerides, which are stored directly in the liver and so used by the body much more quickly than other fats (such as the fats in butter), which are stored in fat cells and so take longer to burn off. Critics, however, view coconut oil much as any other oil – calorie-dense, but unlikely to be harmful if used in small doses.

Melatonin

Melatonin is a natural hormone produced by a small part of the brain called the pineal gland and it is thought to be important in regulating sleep behaviour. It is commercially available and is variously classified in different countries either as a food supplement or, as in Europe, as a drug. It is technically possible for a GP to prescribe it in the UK and it has been used as a sleep promoter, including for children with hyperactivity and for those with 'jet lag'. Studies looking at melatonin output in chronic fatigue syndrome have not shown a deficiency and some have actually shown an increase, so there is no theoretical basis for using it, and despite its popularity melatonin has no convincing evidence to support its use. It does appear to be safe in short-term use, but there is insufficient evidence to say how safe it is when used in the long term. Much as it would be nice to have an effective 'natural' remedy for sleep disturbance, melatonin does not seem to fit the bill.

It may be better to try and get more natural light first thing in the morning, or to use bright light therapy, to try to help to regulate the body's production of melatonin (see p. 35).

Therapeutic massage

Therapeutic massage may be useful in helping people to break out of the grip of stress, and in putting the whole body in a more relaxed state. The deep relaxation it conjures promotes the self-healing response, making room for proper digestion and absorption of nutrients. The heart rate slows and breathing becomes deep instead of shallow (and shallow breathing in itself is calculated to heighten anxiety and tiredness). Therapeutic massage also paves the way for deep, restful sleep, ease aches and pains, improves circulation and increases the overall sense of wellbeing. For people with fibromyalgia, massage may also help with the muscle pain that often characterizes this condition.

Traditional Chinese medicine

Traditional Chinese medicine is one of the oldest forms of health care in the world, going back over 2,500 years. Based on the concept of overall body balance in the form of Yin and Yang, traditional Chinese medicine offers a holistic approach. Symptoms are caused by an imbalance of energy or Qi in a particular meridian. Emotions too can result in illness, especially if they have persisted for a long time or result from stress or trauma. Treatments include acupuncture, herbal medicine, exercise, diet and meditation.

Homoeopathy

Homoeopathy works on the principle that substances harmful in large doses may be beneficial in small doses – roughly like the more modern practice of immunization. While it is best to consult a qualified homoeopath, most pharmacies sell a range of homoeopathic remedies, which may be worth trying first for fatigue. Suggested remedies include:

- zincum metallicum for stress, weakness and exhaustion;
- rhus toxicodendron for muscle fatigue and tiredness;
- arsenicum for restlessness and fatigue accompanied by chills and burning pains that are worse at night; and
- gelsemium for mental exhaustion, including drowsiness and indifference, and for physical weakness, such as heaviness of the limbs and eyelids.

12

Chronic fatigue syndrome, fibromyalgia, candidiasis

These three subjects are grouped together because not only is fatigue a key symptom in them all, but also they are thought to be interlinked and they have many symptoms in common. Some researchers believe that the conditions may be the result of immune dysfunction; others believe that they have to do with hormone imbalances and hypothyroidism.

Whatever the cause, or causes, so similar are their symptoms that you may well be forgiven as to being uncertain as to which condition might be in question. While a doctor can help you make a final diagnosis, some pointers here may be helpful. While fatigue is a common symptom to all, doctors diagnose according to certain differentiating criteria.

- A defining characteristic of fibromyalgia is widespread muscle pain.
- A defining characteristic of chronic fatigue syndrome is fatigue that doesn't improve with rest and that may worsen after physical exertion.
- The defining characteristic of candidiasis isn't so easy to define – as yet there are no firm diagnostic criteria, but characteristics include irritable bowel syndrome and digestive problems, depression and 'brain fog', skin problems and lowered resistance to infection.

Some alternative practitioners have found that all three conditions respond well to an anti-candida diet (see below).

Chronic fatigue syndrome

It's important to realize that feeling tired all the time doesn't necessarily mean you have chronic fatigue syndrome (CFS, also known as myalgic encephalomyelitis, or ME), which is currently recognized as a separate medical condition with certain diagnostic criteria. Classified by the World Health Organization as a disease of the nervous system or neurological disorder, CFS is characterized by prolonged tiredness that does not go away with rest. Characteristically, it is a different type of tiredness from any experienced before, and it isn't linked to lack of drive or motivation as it would be in depression. Sleep tends to be unrefreshing. Fatigue may follow exertion. Muscle and joint pain, headaches, painful lymph nodes and 'brain fog' are among other symptoms.

This kind of long-term, disabling tiredness without a clear medical cause isn't very common. It's difficult to assess the exact prevalence, because studies in different countries have come up with different findings according to how the condition has been defined, but a reasonable average is considered to be around one to two cases per 1,000 people (although many people believe the true incidence to be much higher). It is more common in women than in men.

Several causes or triggers have been suggested for CFS, ranging from the particular, such as infection with the Epstein–Barr virus, to the general, such as the suggestion that CFS may not have one single cause but rather represents the body's response to cumulative physical and emotional stress. Another possible precipitating factor is other infections, particularly ones like influenza, which normally leave a person tired; in this case, for reasons not yet clear, the tiredness persists. As a result there are changes in various hormones and brain chemical transmitters, as well as control mechanisms in the brain that regulate sleep, activity, temperature control and blood pressure. Other triggers may include life stresses such as bereavement, divorce and financial problems. Once CFS is in place, it may be kept going by other, perpetuating factors such as lack of support or poor sleep.

Some studies suggest that a subtle disturbance in brain function may be associated with CFS. New methods of scanning, which highlight active areas of the brain, have revealed differences in the patterns of uptake of glucose (the only fuel that brain tissue can use) in some people with chronic fatigue, although the patterns are not consistent enough to make generalizations.

While we still don't really know what causes and maintains this condition, it is increasingly thought that CFS is an umbrella term for a range of related conditions, and doctors are slowly coming round to acceptance of a physical component in the illness.

While recognition of CFS is comparatively recent – a definition was put together by an international panel of CFS research experts in 1994 – the condition itself appears to have been around for a long time. A textbook from 1750 by English doctor Sir Richard Manningham described 'febricula', or 'little fever', with symptoms very similar to those of CFS, particularly 'great lassitude'. Neurasthenia became a popular diagnosis of the 19th century – it is less popular today, though, because of its psychiatric overtones.

Symptoms and diagnosis

The most common symptom of CFS is an overwhelming feeling of tiredness that is not alleviated by rest, with other medical conditions having been ruled out by the doctor. The tiredness varies from day to day but is present more than half of the time, and when it strikes the tiredness is so disabling as to make it impossible to continue normal physical and mental activities. People may feel too tired to perform normal tasks, or be utterly exhausted for no apparent reason after routine activities or mild exercise. Other symptoms include problems with memory and concentration.

CFS often comes on suddenly, and many people can identify a trigger such as an infection or a stressful experience – again, in the 18th century, Sir Richard Manningham noted its correlation with stress. Many scientists believe that the trigger somehow disrupts the immune system or central nervous system, specifically the hypothalamus–pituitary–adrenal axis – the hypothalamus, pituitary and adrenal glands. These glands affect certain hormones, brain chemical transmitters and control mechanisms in the brain that regulate sleep, activity, temperature control and blood pressure.

In 1994, a panel of international researchers came up with the following criteria for the diagnosis of CFS. They said that for a diagnosis to be made, a person must have had severe chronic fatigue for six months or longer, unrelated to any other known medical conditions, as well as four or more of the following symptoms simultaneously:

- sore throat
- tender lymph nodes
- muscle pain
- diffuse and migratory multi-joint pain without swelling or redness
- headaches of a new type, pattern or severity
- unrefreshing sleep
- aching and listlessness lasting more than 24 hours after exertion.

As stated in Chapter 2, there are many other conditions that may cause CFS-like symptoms, such as anaemia, coeliac disease, liver disease, lupus, multiple sclerosis and thyroid problems, which is why it's important to see your doctor to exclude these as well as conditions such as depression, with which CFS is sometimes confused.

Have I got CFS or am I just tired?

Because tiredness is so common, this question can be a confusing one, but the truth is that, out of all the exhausted many, only a few people are really considered to have CFS. CFS is increasingly recognized as either a specific illness or – perhaps more likely – a group of illnesses that have features in common; indeed, it might be more accurate to call it chronic fatigue *syndromes*.

Symptoms do vary widely among those who have CFS, but, in general, if you have CFS:

- it must be chronic – that is, lasting a long period of time and for at least six months;
- there was probably a definite onset; and
- you must have other symptoms as listed above, such as muscle pain and severe tiredness on minimal exertion.

The main point is that it doesn't go away, even after a few good nights or a holiday.

Getting a diagnosis

A GP will generally be able to diagnose CFS but may wish to have the diagnosis confirmed by a specialist, if one is locally available. Where the GP has made the diagnosis but subsequent progress is slow or the degree of disability very marked, then specialist advice should generally be sought in any case. Only rarely will such a referral reveal some other diagnosis. Potential other benefits of referral include access to more information and local support, specialized services such as physiotherapy or rehabilitation facilities geared towards chronic fatigue and, in a few regions, the possibility of helping with fatigue-related research. There is also benefit in having your case reviewed to ensure that every possible cause of your condition has been looked for and that all available treatments have been tried.

Treatment

Currently, there is no one effective treatment for CFS, but studies have found that people do much better if they remain as active as possible and seek some control over their illness.

A number of drugs are being assessed. These include Ampligen (an antiviral and immune system-modulating drug), modafinil (which is normally used to treat narcolepsy – a daytime sleeping disorder) and low doses of hydrocortisone (because one of the hormonal abnormalities involves a reduced level of cortisol in the blood). Otherwise, drugs are reserved for the symptomatic relief of pain, sleep disturbance and other distressing symptoms. For example, a low dose of a drug called amitriptyline taken shortly before bedtime can be very helpful for pain and sleep disturbance. But medication needs to be used with care as people with CFS are often very sensitive to drugs, particularly those that act on the nervous system.

Managing CFS: set realistic goals

Given the nature of chronic fatigue, many people find it helpful to think in terms of walking before running. For example, you may be very keen to get back to work, but if you are presently off work because of severe chronic fatigue then your first priority is to break down the process of getting back to work into bite-size chunks. That might mean getting back into a routine of waking at the required time and getting up washed and dressed, nothing more. Only once you are able to do that would it be worth going to the next step, which might be coping with travelling to work or regaining a skill that has declined while you have been off work.

You may need to take the advice of family, friends or your doctor at this point in order to keep you realistic.

Cognitive behaviour therapy

In a very under-researched field, cognitive behaviour therapy (CBT) is known to be one of the most successful treatments for CFS, and several studies have shown it to be effective. CBT is the main example of the behavioural treatments, and the theory underlying it is that our reactions to illness depend to an extent on our attitudes and beliefs, which in turn affect our behaviour to illness. This may help or hinder our ability to cope with that illness. The purpose of treatment in this area is to encourage the sort of reactions that help us to deal with being unwell and that promote recovery.

So, why does a psychological therapy help with a physical condition? CBT helps people to identify how their thoughts affect their behaviour. It can help people to develop ways to cope more successfully with fatigue and other symptoms of CFS. The treatment is more effective in milder forms of CFS.

Referral to a psychiatrist for this treatment does not mean that the doctor believes CFS is 'all in the mind'. It is, however, intriguing why a behavioural therapy should be so successful, if, as many posit, chronic fatigue is not a mental disorder but a biological one. A focus on changing beliefs and behaviour is felt by some with CFS to be insulting in view of the evidence for CFS being a physical illness. The implication is taken to be that, as you have 'thought yourself' into being fatigued, so you can 'think yourself' out of it. This is in fact an overly simplistic view of CBT; what the proponents of CBT are saying is that the persistence of illness changes our behaviour in a way that can amplify the symptoms or even create new ones. Behaviour therapists do not say that they can explain why chronic fatigue or any other illness exists, only that they have a system of tackling the effects of illness.

It may be more useful, then, to think in terms of CBT dealing with the effects of long-term illness, or with the symptoms not the cause, and preventing fatigue becoming worse, also in terms of it allowing the self-healing mechanism to take effect. It's also been suggested that CBT has a biological effect, perhaps by helping people to break out of the vicious cycle of the stress response, caused by the stress hormones cortisol and adrenaline (see p. 48), rather than the vicious spiral of beliefs and behaviour that some feel is at the root of fatigue.

The main difficulty with CBT is that it generally must be carried out in conjunction with a trained therapist. Between 10 and 20 one-hour sessions would be the norm, with 'homework' to be done between sessions. The number of NHS therapists (usually psychologists) is small and waiting times of over a year are not uncommon, although the government has invested £170 million towards filling this gap.

How CBT works

The principle is quite simple. First you take a look at some of the attitudes and beliefs that you have about how you feel, and then you look further at the negative ones and re-interpret your attitude in order to try to turn them into something positive. Some examples will illustrate the points more easily.

Let's say that you strongly believe that your fatigue is due to an unknown or undiagnosed physical condition. The 'need to know' creates a block to recovery. Instead, you could try telling yourself that there is certainly a reason for your fatigue, and one of these days it might become obvious, but you haven't got the time to hang about waiting to know what it is. You'll accept, for the meantime at least, that everything reasonable has been done to find a correctable cause for the fatigue, but you'll get on and make the best of things. By accepting the belief that you do not need to know the cause of an illness in order to begin healing from it you have removed the block to improvement.

Often the 'two-column technique' is used to list original beliefs down one side and alternative, more helpful thoughts down the other. For example, see Table 1.

Table 1 The 'two-column technique'

Original view	Alternative view
I'm never going to get better.	Fatigue is unpredictable. I could start improving tomorrow, next week, next year. I still have plenty of interests. I'll focus on one of those.
Exercise only makes me feel worse.	I'm presently coping with as much physical activity as I can handle. After a while I'll try to increase it again. Others have had the same experience.
I'm annoyed that my doctor says I'm depressed and that's why I'm tired.	I've thought it over and really don't feel depressed. I will discuss it with him again.
I'm shattered all the time and get no benefit from sleep.	Although I'm still tired after sleeping, I've done what I can do make it as restful as possible. This is a known problem with chronic fatigue.
No one understands how I feel with this illness.	CFS affects up to 200,000 people in the UK alone. There are lots of good support groups, including many on the internet. I can share my experiences and get support. I can probably help someone else who feels as I do.
My doctor doesn't take me seriously.	Guidelines on diagnosing and managing chronic fatigue conditions are now available to all doctors. I am entitled to a second opinion. I don't need anyone's permission to change my doctor if I want to.
I will lose my job.	CFS is a valid reason to be off work. I have been a good employee and can keep working. I will find out about changing my work patterns to help me cope better.

This may be easier if you can get someone else to help you. Others will probably spot points that you might not notice so easily on your own, or think of alternative reactions to difficult situations. Despite its simplicity this sort of technique can have a strong impact on the experience of illness.

For a detailed, practical approach to using CBT for chronic fatigue, read *Coping with Chronic Fatigue* by Trudie Chalder (Sheldon Press, 2002).

Fibromyalgia

Fibromyalgia, or fibromyalgia syndrome (FMS for short), is a condition characterized by widespread pain in the muscles, tendons, ligaments and nerves. The pain may be felt as achiness or tenderness, especially around the joints, or as tingling or even burning sensations. One feature of the pain is that it may migrate around the body for no apparent reason, although sometimes unaccustomed exercise or movements may cause extra sensitivity.

Fatigue is a prominent symptom, as are sleep problems. Other symptoms include anxiety, irritable bowel syndrome, headaches, morning stiffness, and problems and difficulties with short-term memory and concentration. Fibromyalgia is liable to flare-ups, and symptoms may be exacerbated by factors such as cold or stress. It affects mainly women, and is estimated to affect some 10 per cent of the population.

Many people with hypothyroidism also suffer from fibromyalgia, and some experts believe that it is a variant of thyroid disorder; others point to an immune dysfunction as being the root of both disorders.

Treatment usually consists of a combination of antidepressant medication, psychotherapy and gentle exercise. Research has shown that exercise can significantly improve the symptoms of fibromyalgia for most people, reducing pain, boosting energy levels and helping with regular sleep patterns. Low-impact aerobic exercises – such as walking, cycling or swimming – are thought to be best, rather than muscle-straining exercises such as weight-training. The right diet may also be very helpful. There is advice below and in Chapter 9, but for a thorough look at the subject, do read *The Fibromyalgia Healing Diet* by Christine Craggs-Hinton (Sheldon Press, 2008).

Candida albicans

In recent years, *Candida albicans* has been closely implicated with fatigue in general, and with CFS in particular, as well as with other conditions including thrush, abdominal bloating, depression, poor resistance to infection, irritable bowel syndrome, unexpected weight gain, difficulty in concentrating and cravings for sugar or alcohol.

Candida albicans is a fungus or yeast normally present in the bowel; it is nourished by simple carbohydrates in our diet such as found in sugar, bread, biscuits and cakes. In its normal small amounts it is harmless and kept under control by friendly bacteria in the gut, but it is believed to grow out of control in certain conditions (candidiasis). Conditions conducive to candidiasis include a diet high in sugary foods and refined carbohydrates (like white bread, cakes, biscuits and pasta); a diet high in fermented foods, such as cheese, alcohol, vinegar and pickles; repeat courses of antibiotics; the use of hormone replacement therapy or the contraceptive pill; and prolonged periods of stress. Once grown out of control, the *Candida* fungus is believed to release wastes into the bloodstream that affect the nervous system and immune system, creating a wide variety of symptoms.

While conventional medical practice tends to view yeast problems as primarily thrush, many alternative practitioners believe that untreated intestinal candidiasis that has spread through the body may be a prime cause of chronic fatigue syndrome. When the *Candida* fungus releases wastes into the body, this is thought to create a variety of symptoms. As well as persistent tiredness, other symptoms of candidiasis include skin infections, allergies, abdominal bloating, poor resistance to infection, irritable bowel syndrome, unexpected weight gain and cravings for sugar or alcohol, allergies, depression, headaches, irritability, difficulties in concentrating and memory loss.

Candida is thought to be a major reason why some people cannot lose weight despite their best efforts. Cravings for sugar and bread are certainly not the best foundation for healthy weight. Some people find that they benefit – and lose significant weight – when they stop eating grains altogether, especially wheat, and add more protein to their diet to help to keep blood sugar levels stable. Cravings for simple carbohydrates such as found in bread, biscuits and cakes are thought by many alternative practitioners to be masked food allergy, causing a kind of 'addiction' in people to the very foods to which they are sensitive.

Candidiasis is hard to diagnose by conventional medical means, but one way to is to look at your diet and your symptoms. If you crave sugar, bread or other carbohydrates, are experiencing any other symptoms or just don't feel well, you may benefit from the following dietary suggestions.

- Eat vegetables.
- Eat enough proteins, such as found in fish and other lean meats. Try including some protein with every meal. This helps to boost your metabolism and keep your blood sugar levels stable.
- Avoid carbohydrates, sugars and alcohol.
- Avoid fermented foods such as alcohol, cheese, smoked fish and meats, and sausages.
- Avoid yeast products and mushrooms.
- For a while, avoid fruit and fruit juices since they contain concentrated fructose, a natural fruit sugar that may feed the *Candida*.

- Eat only small amounts of dairy products because they contain lactose, a milk sugar.
- Ensure you keep your blood sugar levels up by eating a substantial breakfast, lunch and dinner, with snacks if necessary.
- Drink plenty of water.

After a few days of this, some of your symptoms may become worse and you could also experience headaches (the so-called 'die-off' reaction as the body adjusts to giving up foods to which it is accustomed). Prepare yourself also for strong cravings for bread, cakes and sweets; alternative practitioners say that *Candida* thrives on sugar and simple carbohydrates and doesn't give up its treats easily! Cravings may be helped by small regular amounts of protein. Any adverse reactions should improve after a few days, at which point you can expect to start feeling better.

After a week or so, you may slowly add fresh fruits, to be eaten by themselves, and on an empty stomach. Fruit is very easily digested and moves through the body quickly. However, if it is eaten with a heavier food like protein, fat or starch, the sugary fruit will remain in the stomach until the heavier food is broken down and then ferments in the stomach, thus making the problem worse (which is thought to be why many people with *Candida* have problems eating fruit).

Useful addresses and further reading

Useful addresses

UK

Action for M.E.
Third Floor, Canningford House
38 Victoria Street
Bristol BS1 6BY
Tel.: 0845 123 2314 (11a.m. to 1p.m., Monday to Friday; 6.30p.m. to 8.30p.m., Monday)
Website: www.afme.org.uk

Provides support for those with myalgic encephalomyelitis (ME); see also ME Association below.

British Association for Behavioural and Cognitive Psychotherapies
Victoria Buildings
9–13 Silver Street
Bury BL9 0EU
Tel.: 0161 797 4484
Website: www.babcp.com

British Snoring and Sleep Apnoea Association Castle Court
41 London Road
Reigate RH2 9EL
Tel.: 01737 245638
Website: www.britishsnoring.co.uk

Chronic Fatigue Research and Treatment Unit
King's College Hospital
Mapother House
De Crespigny Park
Denmark Hill
London SE5 8AZ
Tel.: 020 3228 5075
Website: kcl.ac.uk/projects/cfs

ME Association
4 Top Angel
Buckingham Industrial Park
Buckingham MK18 1TH
Tel.: 012080 818968 (9.30a.m. to 4.30p.m.)
Website: www.meassociation.org.uk

A cross-party group of Members of Parliament in the UK have produced a report into known of the causes and treatment of CFS/ME. The Gibson Inquiry is available on line at www.erythos.com/gibsonenquiry/docs/ME_Inquiry_Report.pdf

Narcolepsy Association
Website: www.narcolepsy.org.uk

National Candida Society
PO Box 151
Orpington
Kent BR5 1UJ
Tel.: 01689 813 039
Website: www.candida-society.org

Provides information and support to people with candida, and attempts to raise public awareness of the condition.

The Sleep Council
High Corn Mill
Chapel Hill
Skipton
North Yorkshire BD23 1NL
Tel.: 0845 058 4595 (admin)
Freephone Leaflet line: 0800 018 7923
Website: www.sleepcouncil.com

Sleep Matters Medical Advisory
Service
Tel: 020 8994 9874

Thyroid UK
32 Darcy Road
St Osyth
Clacton on Sea
Essex CO16 8QF
Tel.: 01255 820407 (permanent
answerphone)
Website: www.thyroiduk.org

USA

The Chronic Fatigue Association
of America
P.O. Box 220398
Charlotte
NC 28222-0398
Tel.: 704 365 2343
Website: www.cfids.org

Sleepless in America
Depression and Bipolar Support
Alliance
730 N. Franklin Street, Suite 501
Chicago
IL 60610-7224
Tel.: 800 826 3632
Website: www.sleeplessinamerica.org

Further reading

M. Burgess and T. Chalder (2005) *Overcoming Chronic Fatigue*, Robinson Publishing.

F. Campling and M. Sharpe (2008) *Chronic Fatigue Syndrome: The facts*, Oxford University Press.

T. Cantopher (2006) *Depressive Illness: The Curse of the Strong*, Sheldon Press.

T. Chalder (2002) *Coping with Chronic Fatigue*, Sheldon Press.

C. Craggs-Hinton (2003) *The Chronic Fatigue Healing Diet*, Sheldon Press.

J. Horne (2006) *Sleepfaring: A Journey Through the Science of Sleep*, Oxford University Press.

I. Gibson, *Inquiry into the Status of CFS/ME and Research into Causes and Treatment* (2006) The Group on Scientific Research into Myalgic Encephalomyelitis (ME) (A report produced by a cross-party committee of UK MPs: <http://www.erythos.com/gibsonenquiry/Docs/ME_Inquiry_Report.pdf>).

N. Read (2006) *Sick and Tired: Healing the Illnesses that Doctors Cannot Cure*, Orion.

M. Sharpe and D. Wilks (2002) Fatigue, *British Medical Journal*, vol. 325, pp.480–3 (<http://www.bmj.com/cgi/content/full/325/7362/480>).

R. Wiseman (2007) *Quirkology: The Curious Science of Everyday Lives*, Macmillan.

J. Worthington, A. Fletcher and C. Collins (2007) *The Duvet Diet: Sleep Yourself Slim*, Rodale.

Index